GIVING VOIC
INNER SC

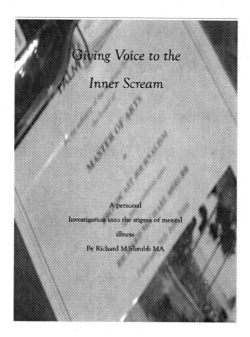

Giving Voice to the

Inner Scream

A personal
Investigation into the stigma of mental
illness
By Richard M Shrubb MA

RICHARD SHRUBB

'One million people commit suicide every year'
The World Health Organization

RICHARD SHRUBB

Published by
Chipmunkapublishing
PO Box 6872
Brentwood
Essex CM13 1ZT
United Kingdom

http://www.chipmunkapublishing.com

GIVING VOICE TO THE INNER SCREAM

To all those who may doubt us:

If you doubt yourself at your lowest point when all around you is wrong, then look at yourself when you recover your ability to forge ahead with life.

We are just the same.

RICHARD SHRUBB

Why write this book?

"Pissed weirdo seeks work. Have a vocational degree in maritime business and want to earn a living without looking at a ship again. £30 000 a good salary, happy to work in a call centre. Temper unpredictable, am under stress from not knowing anything about this world except from my international and public school upbringing, and have no friends in this city. Have to take every other Wednesday off as am in Court in Southampton. References might come in from my moneyed Godfather and a CIA officer in the US who oversaw my time on a sailing ship as I got pissed and laid in the Midwest about 5 years back. Someone pay me this money as I am intelligent..."

Such might have been written a "job wanted" advert back in 1997 when I finally faced the real world for the first time, aged 23.

Contrast this to someone tapped on the shoulder at a press event by an international news agency some 7 years later:

"MA in broadcast journalism from a top university. Prior education on 2 continents and several islands in the university of life, with a degree in maritime business. In depth knowledge of US and UK politics, and a working knowledge of European culture. A passion for world affairs, consume several hours of news a week."

This is the same man. Irony? I earned around £20 000 a year when in the first job advert and wound up jobless, homeless and in survival mode because of the second. Why? I have a diagnosis of paranoid schizophrenia and know I shouldn't drink again.

Indeed, the pages you read are the culmination of some 5 years work toward making a living as a journalist. I won't be paid for a year after you read this, and will get a very small percentage of the book you buy. (Buy one for a friend!). Life has taught me a lesson – the stigma of mental illness is more disabling than the illness itself.

In this chapter, I start with a rundown of the life and career that led to writing this book, then I'll look at the chapters written that succeed it. The book is about the stigma of mental illness, in this chapter you'll see what I am getting at the better.

+++
++++++++++++++++++++++++++++++

I was born to a Royal Naval Officer and a Computer Manager in Portsmouth in 1974. Thomas Harris relates in his books how Hannibal Lecter travels through memory in a "memory palace" – I travel through my years by going to places in which I lived.

Thus Portsmouth became Plymouth became Waterlooville became Terfuren became Stoke Climsland became Virginia Beach became Stoke Climsland....

GIVING VOICE TO THE INNER SCREAM

I was multilingual in Terfuren, a Flemish suburb of Brussels. Had to, a first sink or swim moment for me was going to a kindergarten where no one spoke English. With no Flemish speakers willing to teach Dad, so I translated for him. He had NATO friends who were German and half of Brussels was French so he taught me the basics of those languages too!

A summer holiday in those days involved Mum and I following Dad to a NATO conference by road somewhere else in Europe. Consequently we drove to Pisa, Geneva, and Bonne.

War broke out in the Falklands, delaying our posting to the US by 6 months. Dad fought the war hard, sleeping on the barracks steps on Ascension Island and making sure squaddies had at least one toothbrush per unit in his guise of supplies officer on the QE2.

So, amid dreams of snakes and the movie *Jaws*, which had recently come out on TV, we flew to Virginia Beach, Virginia. Dad fought the Cold War from a desk in Norfolk VA, getting Duty Free supplies of booze from the mess for Mum to throw wild parties with.

I was a delinquent, and managed to get expelled from the local Kingston Elementary School after 18 months for not doing homework. Not having a school to go to, this coincided with my American friends being posted elsewhere, David Shea to

San Diego and Andy Brown to Boston. Dad kept his posting in Norfolk and moved house from Kings Grant to a beach front apartment in Va Beach proper. I however got my marching orders and went to prep school in Barnstaple, North Devon. This meant a 4000 mile commute to school by jumbo jet and train, three times a year, each way.

Hated the place. It was just too far from home. Given the choice between a school of stuffed shirts and a beachfront apartment, what would you choose? My memories of those days are of the holidays, one on a sailing ship that Dad had a lecture junket on from Jamaica to Bermuda, and another driving from LA via the Grand Canyon to San Francisco. Now, a snow covered hole in the ground (the Grand Canyon) against chilblains and snobbery at a piss hole in the North Devon snow...? David Cassell, the headmaster, was later convicted for paedophilia, sums things up really.

Mum and Dad were having difficulties. Serious ones, not only from having a delinquent 10 year old living 4000 miles away. I first heard the word "divorce" in the 70's. 12 years after the marriage started, so it broke up in Cornwall, I at school and even more stressed about Cornwall as a home than Va Beach.

Dad got a posting in the Falklands, this time living in a Portacabin in Stanley. Made it to the war zone in the end! He had the wonderful acronym of PSO CBFFI. Personal Service Officer to Commanding

GIVING VOICE TO THE INNER SCREAM

Officer, British Forces Falkland Islands. Secretary to the boss.

I flew out that Christmas, this time given the choice between the Falkland Islands and a high street flat in Bromyard. Mum lost her son again, this time made the worse when I enjoyed Christmas so much I stayed for New Year. Her first "single" festive season more single than even she imagined it would.

A romance developed in a blizzard that southern hemisphere autumn. Dad was given penicillin for an illness, and he was allergic. Naked, windows open and still overheating, so Dr Josephine Kingston gave him the antidote. He married her 2 years later.

My next posting was given that summer, and I went to the Royal Hospital School where I was to become an alcoholic and be guaranteed mental illness. Oh yeah, 7 C's and a B at GCSE and 3 E's at A level.

I was there for 6 years. The school's greatest achievement in my opinion was its clock tower being a navigation aid to the Luftwaffe in World War 2. Treasonous and duplicitous, the two things ingrained into any free thinker that had the misfortune to be incarcerated there. Treason and duplicity, the school was for the sons of the Royal Navy Lower Deck and by that I mean the bilges where the rats daren't tread. So by providing an education to this lot in such finery, it became a navigation aid for the mass murder of Londoners in World War 2.

By this time an alcoholic and heavy smoker, as well as having about 9 more addresses to my name, I went to the US to work on a sailing ship for two seasons. I look back to that year as one of sadness and difficulty. I hadn't lived in the real world for 8 years so didn't know what real people were like. All home addresses had been transitory and I had stayed for maybe 5 months a year there, or should I say "theres". I then went to school for 7 months a year where I was a reject – I was a caged animal when finally let out at sea. I was on a sailing ship with an alcohol problem and fire fighting my way from immigration problems to women's knickers-elastic problems to drunken brawls in ghettos. I saw some fine sights though, did some wicked things... How many Brits can say they have walked half a mile onto a Great Lake in winter and stood watch in the very same spot that summer on a 200 ft sailing ship?!

Still confused and angry at the world, so I returned to the UK to go on the dole for a summer and get wrecked at the homes of school friends. A jobless bum on marijuana, at least then I had a degree to go on that October, 1994. I discovered LSD, psilocybin mushrooms, Ecstasy and amphetamines. Five addresses in 3 years....

So I did my degree in the University of Life and Southampton's polytechnic. I got a First Class in paranoid schizophrenia and a Third Class in

GIVING VOICE TO THE INNER SCREAM

Maritime Studies. I also nearly got time in prison from a woman who hated men and decided that prison was the place I needed to go to "become a man". I got out of Southampton in the hope my problems would stay there…

I had good looks, a 32 inch waist and 42 inch chest. I was worldly. All I needed was a job and a career and a social life. Firstly, I needed to learn about the Real World. So Dad evicted me from my house in Fishponds in Bristol and told me to go to the Salvation Army. Always different, I went to the Youth Hostel in the centre of town. I temped rather than went on the dole, and at one stage for 50 hours a week was on about £20 Grand Pre tax. Still failed to pay my rent and was pissed most of the time on that. In this way I weirded out every employment agency in Bristol.

Jobs got farther apart and more difficult to get. "Don't you know who I am?" I screamed at the world… Silence, the world blanking me in the way someone affronted would deny you response in the supermarket. The inner scream was silent, only now do I give voice to it in the book of that name.

I had an ace up my sleeve. I was experiencing something that I decided to reveal to my father. I believe that when I speak to my stereo, people listening to the radio station I am tuned into can hear my voice (I still do). In my opinion I was a radio pirate. I had been experiencing this for about 3 years but never shared it, except through the radio, with anyone[1]. So a secret radio pirate at home, I did not let on to anyone outside my mind. I was in a fix, unemployable and unemployed, angry and incapable of making friends, and friendless.

Dad tricked me into telling my GP about it, and I was referred up to the mental health services where I negotiated a spell at Southmead Hospital's day care unit. Shortly, a social worker visited my bed-sit and she decided that I should move to a shared house for psychiatric patients in the centre of Bristol.

Though my position in society plummeted from "slightly weird, good looking bloke" to "dribbling nutter" my life significantly improved. I was awarded Disability Living Allowance and had an income of £170 a week and my rent paid on top of that. Even though I cried buckets at my label of "schizophrenic" things were really getting better. I had friends, and I started to find my way into journalism. My best friend Emily, whom I had met in Virginia in the mid 80's, told me I was a good writer so I did a correspondence course. This course led to a writing circle where I wrote 150 000 words for three chapters on my life at sea (the book you're reading is about 45 000). I then did an A Level equivalent at City of Bristol College in journalism. I was encouraged by Bob Pitt, my tutor, to apply to Falmouth College of Arts to do a Post Graduate Diploma in broadcast journalism.

---

[1] A full explanation of the symptoms is found in the next chapter

GIVING VOICE TO THE INNER SCREAM

I was still a practising alcoholic, and this did not stop. I took a year out between college and university to sort my head out before doing the PG Dip. Nothing changed. I then moved house to Cornwall.

From a house of hedonistic headcases, so I moved to a shared house of students. I was the chief hedonist, pubbing until the money ran out and then borrowed on credit card. I have one person to mention in that house, a 19 year old dance student. At the outset I told the landlady that I didn't want a 19 year old in my house because of an incident where a 30 year old had cracked my 19 year old university friend's skull with a chair back in Southampton. 19 year olds are too old to live in a 30 year old's house for the reason that they are too old to live at home with their parents. In part we did not get on because I was 30, in a large part we did not get on because she was 19.

The drink became an issue not because I was friendless and incapable of making friends, so much as I had made friends with Kirsty Hemming and her friend Dena Tahmesebi. I basically got tangled up in their affairs and was about to be thrown off the course when I won my negotiations to be put on the anti alcohol drug Antabuse. Antabuse was at this time implanted in the ex footballer George Best's stomach and its reaction with his renewed alcoholism killed him. I have knowingly consumed alcohol one time since and got violent diarrhoea from a Coffee Liqueur ice cream.

So, Kirsty in her attempts to get the stalking Richard Shrubb out of her life, changed his for the better. I thanked her at a party at the end of the academic year, when I would go on to do a thesis and upgrade the PG Dip into a Master's Degree. Shortly after sobering up I was at a press event with Press Association when I got tapped on the shoulder by a news agency.

I was interviewed later that summer and told that they would very much like me aboard. A week of waiting and no contract arriving in the post, I left a message on their voice mail saying that I get very paranoid and was this offer too good to be true? They phoned up, asking what I meant by paranoia, and I explained that I have psychosis.

I was due to go house hunting in London that week, my tenancy at Windsor Terrace was due to end the week after that. I was told I had been aggressive on the phone and they were withdrawing their job offer. In short, they saw more acutely the label I have than the CV that they had on their desk.

Suing them under the Disability Discrimination Act, I had to move and fast to not be homeless, so to a flat in St Pauls in Bristol paid for on credit card. I was then bound to live there under UK tenancy law for 6 months, or on giving two months' notice. What employer would take you on with 2 months' notice given every Jade Goody in the world wants the same job? I was fucked in short.

The news agency said they'd fight their case and my legal funding ran out so I had to withdraw my lawsuit. No one would back me through the courts – not even the Disability Rights Commission.

I have had to think on my feet and make drastic decisions at the shot of a gun in my time. I am expert in it. This time I would refuse to carry on like that. A friend was running a Restricted Service Licence radio station so I made a half hour documentary on the history of psychiatric treatment to Isambard Brunel's death (he wasn't nutty, he was just being remembered in Bristol to 2006)[2]. I met someone who agreed to mentor me writing a book and with my career as a freelance journalist. Toby oversaw me getting the sample chapter of this book together amid a Lottery bid to set up a radio station for Bristol psychiatric patients. The bid refused, I won this publishing deal.

After a 9 year break from successful romance, I met a wonderful woman and am deeply in love with her. In a "Hayes Daze" this book is written.

The cry of "I don't deserve this shit" was heard and people employed me until I showed them I was nuts. I then proved that I was due a better life by recovering from mental illness and this

---

[2] You can hear it here www.b200fm.com/lunacy.htm, 25 minutes in length.

recovery has made me labelled so that even though my qualifications make me eminently more employable than before, I am doubly more unemployable than I was because of the label "schizophrenic". Go figure!

++ +++++++++++++++++++++++++++++++++++

Here is a précis of the book. I am not the only person to lose in the face the stigma of mental illness. I met a guy who committed murder because of mental illness so faces a struggle in rehabilitation that I thankfully don't even have to contemplate.. The chapter is named after the anonymous "psycho killer", *Andrew*. Andrew is a down to earth, calm guy who doesn't take drugs except those prescribed him. Of the many people I have met with mental illness, I hold this man as one of the best, solid, decent of men to have been referred to the system. To my mind, if you can look Andrew in the eye and say what I have just said, you cannot attach the psycho killer label to me and use that label to make him, or me, unemployable.

I went through a mental process in meeting Andrew. I was at first afraid (as anyone who knew of murder committed by another man). I girded my loins and visited him. He lived in a shared house for psychiatric patients in Bristol. I found what I described above, and in so doing, had to challenge my own perceptions of mental illness.

GIVING VOICE TO THE INNER SCREAM

It inspired me. If I had to go through this journey, what would your Middle Englander have to do to achieve the same? For the people who would read this text, people who are interested in challenging the stigma of mental illness, hopefully you will challenge your own perceptions of mental illness yourself, even the more educated and least likely to label amongst you. Read and understand, due to the lies of a diseased mind, a good man can be led to murder…

In *Safety Net* I then look at the supported housing system that enabled him to reacquaint with the world. *Supporting People* is a £2 billion scheme that is designed to protect the tenancies of, and support the daily challenges of living in society of people who have been disabled from doing so for a variety of reasons. I lived in supported accommodation for 5 years, and went on from being a loser in every sense of the word, to an MA and then onto a publishing deal. Andrew has an ambition. To do a day's work, stop off at the pub for a soft drink on the way home and fuck his wife at the end of the day. Straight out of Rampton he'd face what two of his former fellow interns at Rampton and Broadmoor (in the chapter *The basket weavers and the basket case*) face. He might have been made homeless and exposed to the very factors that sent him crazy in the first place, mental illness and hard drugs as a relief from it all.

Supporting People shocked the government by its success and the cost. The cost shocked it more than the success – an estimated budget of £700 million ended up closer to £2 billion, and the Treasury immediately sought ways of reducing the expenditure and may end up with a third of those receiving support from the scheme in Bristol being thrown out on the streets. They may even find themselves one of the many written about in the final investigation, *Basket weavers*. Why is a scheme, credited with saving £2 for every £1 spent on supported housing, facing cuts? This chapter seeks answers from the government after finding out the extent to which dithering and silence is affecting the management of these houses.

The next chapter is called *A mad world*. World famous hedonist, drugs fiend and journalist Hunter S Thompson committed suicide in 2005. He blew his brains out with a Magnum pistol in front of his son. Up to then he was famous the world over for his drug fuelled exploits and high jinx. In his memoirs, *Kingdom of Fear* he related how an ageing ex hippy asked him, *how did you survive the Sixties and continue in this way through the turn of the century?*

My answer has changed since his suicide. He did not survive. In the instant that his hand squeezed the trigger of his high powered handgun he changed from a model hell raising citizen, to a mentally disordered man who killed himself because of his illness.

GIVING VOICE TO THE INNER SCREAM

I suggest that the reader should consume some of his works before reading this chapter. Only then do you have the moral right to go through the journey of seeing a man lauded for hedonism as nothing but a mentally ill suicide victim. I asked a psychiatrist for diagnoses of his illnesses, and ended up not diagnosing Hunter S Thompson but the tribes of hedonists who turn British city centres into war zones on a Friday night. What's a saner place on a Friday night at midnight, the Lime Unit in Callington Rd Hospital or Bristol's Centre?

I then look at the humble heroin addict in *Junky*. This group of people is stigmatised in the media on a daily basis because of their love of a drug that makes daily living seem possible and worthwhile to them. Heavily referring to *The Heroin Addicts* by Tam Stewart, I compare the life of the tea drinker to the nicotine addict to the alcoholic to the junky. The sentence preceding has a gradient from the tea drinker at the top of society to the junky at the perceived bottom. I am going to level that line, arguing that the lowest of the low is not the junky but the man who judges the junky. I also give an underhand compliment to George Best (the dead footballer)...

What's so wonderful about sticking a needle in your arm despite the correct stigmatisation of the drug in a world where from the age of 6 everyone knows that heroin is a nasty addiction?

The basket weavers and the basket case deals with the homeless mentally ill. The Salvation Army

Hostel in Bristol is a welcome refuge from the rigours of polydrug addiction and street life. Yet these people have a steep hill to climb even if they are lucky enough to win a roof over their heads at the hostel. Generally mentally ill and with two or more chemical addictions the care systems in place seem not to want to give these men help.

Even if the hostel secures them an assessment by the mental health authorities, they are generally referred on to drug misuse authorities and then back to the mental health system. If the wrangling is silenced, and this is not often, there is generally another problem. Many are addicted to benzodiazepines such as Lorazepam and Valium. Prescribed these drugs by a doctor for their mental health issues, they can buy the pills down the pub for £2 a pill, so become addicted. Then the Salvation Army has difficulty, it will not detoxify people addicted to benzos because they may hide mental health problems that can be exacerbated by coming off the prescription drugs.

Welcome to a steep slippery sided pit where people cannot always help you to get out. I seek answers from the Avon and Wiltshire Partnership mental health NHS Trust. Just what is going on for a regular event such as the homeless mentally ill drug abuser to be consistently passed from pillar to post, in the apparent hope that they will just go away and not seek treatment? I raise a withering attack on AWP, justified in my opinion because through institutional "games of tennis" some of the most vulnerable people in society fall through the net of the Welfare State. This is unforgivable and should be remedied.

+++
++++++++++++++++++++++++++++++++++++

My girlfriend wonders at my frequent dalliance with drugs in this book. Very little, it will be seen, leaves the realms of narcotics for long. She cracked up under strain alone, and is teetotal with her religion. Many people suffer, whether the executive from stress, to the teenager who hears voices from a young age and never stops.

Mental illness is caused, as a car hitting your leg causes that leg to be broken. In my experience of mental illness and the people suffering it, there is generally a car wreck of sorts in their lives, and their minds are broken. I write this whilst sure that BBC 6 Music's Steve Lamacq can hear my keystrokes as I type. Though people recover to the point that they can function and operate in the normal world, very few walk away completely unscathed.

Celebrities. The religion of the masses in Twenty First Century Britain. More know the life history of the DJ Chris Moyles than the demise of the Turkish Caliphate and the causation of Bush's civil war in Iraq. I mention the celebrities in question throughout this book because people feel they know them and, in seeing their mental illness, I hope you will see a readily accessible person of illness that you might not otherwise know. Which

Irishman didn't know of George Best, and, if not you'll know him if you fly via Belfast's main airport! Hunter S Thompson and even Robbie Williams take the stage in this works. They all have problems and are symptomatic of society in general – you know someone with mental illness even if you read the red top papers every day, never mind knowing a cigarette smoker (who I compare to the heroin addict).

Equally, how many people don't know of the war zone that erupts in your city centre on a Friday night, and of the mental illnesses that are simulated in the midst of mass hysteria and alcohol mania? By saying every 21 year old in a short skirt, barfing on the pavement is mentally ill at the time, you will realise that the stigma is pointless by virtue it should be applied to 90% of the UK population, not to the 1% with a diagnosis.

In my travels for writing this book, I came upon an eminent professor who used a big word that sums up what I intend to do with this book. Using my experience and knowledge of the stigma of mental illness firsthand, he said that I am trying to "demystify" mental illness. By removing the myth of a dribbling psycho or the needle jabbing junky and exposing the man beneath, I hope to dispel the media myths around which society considers its judgements on people within. I hope you will see the man or the animal beneath. Andrew the man, the projectile vomiting pisshead in the centre of town on Friday night, the animal. Good luck!

GIVING VOICE TO THE INNER SCREAM

Andrew

My friends were nervous. Dark rumours abounded of a psychopathic knifeman moving into a half way house in Bristol. I was at university in Cornwall, studying for my Masters degree. My group of friends had known mental illness for what it really is; a disabling condition. We only affected people outside of our inner lives by acting weird or shutting ourselves away; a more typical incident happening at my shared house in 2000 where after a 6 month decline, one of us was eventually Sectioned for self neglect.

Matt was tormented with his voices, and extremely scared of leaving the house; a term we called "paranoid", or irrational fear. Many people reading this will have heard of agoraphobia. So because of paranoia, Matt had agoraphobia, and couldn't get out even to do his food shopping. Perhaps you should then add hydrophobia because the man did not wash for six months. To us this meant a smelly, weak man who would collapse if he stood to answer the front door because his blood sugar levels were so low. What does this form of mental illness mean to society? Unless we as a house and the staff had not intervened, a corpse would have been carried out one day; as was, not even that. Matt made zero impact on society because he was so withdrawn from it.

Andrew's arrival blew the doors open for us. Even among the highs and lows of a group of schizophrenic friends, murder (unlike suicide) was an unknown quantity for us; it was something that *they* did, *they* being people who wound up in the whispered about hospitals of Ashworth, Rampton and Broadmoor. *They*, Hannibal Lecter, Peter Sutcliffe.

I heard through the grapevine that Andrew was sober and hated people smoking cannabis, something that I had banned from my house because it does people of our past no good at all. When I was in supported accommodation I was a practising alcoholic. Consequently, because of me it had the ups and downs of a man struggling with drink and the people in his surrounds struggling with their own problems – and mine. My mate was nervous when during one of my visits from Falmouth, I decided to meet him round at Andrew's house.

I warmed to him immediately. Happy people lead happy lives, depressed and struggling people lead depressing and struggling lives. The house was of the former, though no doubt by its very nature a place where people were concerned about making their way out of a much demeaned and stigmatised world. I returned to Bristol in 2005, Andrew helping me move to a flat in St Paul's. Of the pair of us, this man is the nicer man. Why? I pondered. I took to having coffee with him on a regular basis, monthly chats getting wired at a favourite local coffee shop. Why look up to a man who had freaked out and stabbed people?

The answer lies in the question. For him to be let out of secure accommodation he had to pass the personality test. In the case of people confined "at Her Majesty's Pleasure" to a secure psychiatric hospital, there is only one way to get out, to be well. I have not met anyone who has killed because of rational reasons and "done life" (military men, yes). One would hazard that after "doing life" in the prison system the killer is released because he has served the time the judge told him to. It is implicit in the conditions that most people are sent to Broadmoor or Rampton that these people have to pass a variety of psychological tests before they're even considered for release. Andrew, in short, is of sounder mind than I because if he was not, he would not be having coffee with me and still be detained at Her Majesty's Pleasure.

We might compare the retired military man, who has killed on duty, with the man who has killed whilst ill. The retired officer or grunt, both of whom I have known, is placid to the point of softness. The serving soldier I knew, a Commando, was very safe at home, you were completely at ease with him. However you sensed that there was something far more alert, like electricity flowing. The feeling elicited is of "a good man, but by God I'm glad I won't be at the opposite end of the battlefield from him". Andrew has the gentility of the retired military man. One who could, knows he can, but has switched it off for good, and will entertain any length to never go there again. Here is a man who had done his crime, served his time, yet despite having done what turned out to be something quite minor as murders go, is likely to serve another life sentence *at society's pleasure* because he was not clinically responsible for the act he committed.

Over three interviews with Andrew I recorded his story. Andrew said what follows.

I was born in Yorkshire. My earliest memory is of Dad buying a colour telly and bringing his mates round every weekend to get pissed and watch Match of the Day. I grew up thinking that this is not the way I want to be, ignoring us kids. When I was 7, Mum met a guy who lived in Essex in the pub she worked at, and eventually moved to Essex with the bloke who would become my step dad. I respected him more than my father because he took notice of us. Because of him I had a good, stable childhood.

I went to a few schools up North and a number of primary schools in Essex because my parents were moving around. I wasn't expelled or anything. At some point when I was at school, I wanted to start earning money, so got a job down the market selling fruit and veg. I done that for about 3 years - £20 a day and going to school. I sometimes truanted to go to work. When I was 16 I got a job at an off license, three jobs and school – I was no sponge! Got my GCSE's, did 7 exams... I wasn't the brightest kid but I was earning so what did it matter?

What did matter was a day when my best mate visited me at the office. He went home and got electrocuted mowing the lawn, the shock killing him instantly. I see this as the reason everything went wrong in the end, blaming myself since if he hadn't visited he wouldn't have gone home and died. I was the only friend of his to turn up to the funeral. My mates and I used to get beer from my work and take "medication" to get pissed like kids of that age do but with my friend gone I started to drink heavily. I was angry and found that booze and drugs made things feel better, yet pissed I was even angrier. I have memories of turning up home at 3 in the morning and my parents refusing to let me in. My neighbours noticed me sleeping in the garden, not good.

Aged 16 and schooldays finished, I got a job as an apprentice tool maker at Marconi Avionics. The money was good and so were the prospects but let's face it, factory work isn't for everyone. My uncle got me a job fitting air conditioning after 9 months and I quit the apprenticeship. Good times they were, working Monday to Friday, London at the weekends with my mates to get shitfaced. You know what its like; get your money, go out, get lathered, wake up with random women – [surprised] "I didn't did I?!" Sometimes waking up early in the morning on the Central Line tube at the end of the line, no way of getting home!

The first time I went to prison I was lodging with three others in a house in Chelmsford. All of us were alcoholics feeding off each other. "I'll never drink again… oh alright I'll have one with you since you're offering". One day I was arrested for shoplifting whisky and wine at the supermarket… I was in the police cells when they found the landlord drowned in the bath. The other two were arrested for a double killing because the police thought they'd done me in as well. I was arrested in the dock at the Magistrates after a few weeks on remand for the shoplifting, for manslaughter. I was on remand for 9 months going through the court process. At Crown Court all three of us were acquitted.

Life was colourful after that spell in the nick. There was a three year waiting list for council housing even if you were homeless so, having been kicked out of my parents' house before I was jailed, I was sleeping on sofas. A mate was on a video round, delivering videos as rental. He and I got it in our heads to sell them on street corners. We used the money to get pissed. Stealing booze or other things… A great way to get breakfast, I found, was to get arrested. If you had Magistrates' in the morning the police would have to feed you. You'd also get a doctor's appointment in there as well and be put on anti alcohol craving or detox pills. For whatever reason I'd get 28 days here, 3 months there… I lost count of the amount of time I spent inside or how many spells I got. Shoplifting, drunk and disorderly, non payment of fines…

People on the outside didn't understand why I liked it in there but if you knew the system you'd do alright. I found that prison was an easier life than that outside, like a hotel! Three meals a day and if you got a job, you got paid so could afford tobacco. There was routine, rules to follow, and regular meals. You couldn't really want for more with life outside as hard as it was.

++++++++

Prospects[3] is a new project run by the Home Office whose aim is to take people in Andrew's situation in the late 1980's, and to show them a way of living that is more rewarding[4]. If there was something like this for Andrew, would it have changed him? Andrew's response that it is a rhetorical question with no answer. *"How do I know, there weren't anything like that for me?"*

Rarely for a current government criminal project, this is about rehabilitating people in this situation, tackling a major economic headache without New Labour's habitual constriction of rights but a positive, carrot based approach. It is a scheme of supported housing for repeat drugs offenders who are stuck in the cycle of needing crime to feed their drugs habits and taking prison as an occupational hazard. The aim is straightforward – to provide a Petri dish in which drug offenders may catch the habits and experience the rewards of the norm. Three meals a day is not ordinary for these people, let alone the settled feeling one gets at the end of the day after work and a bellyful of good food. Andrew needed £25 worth of alcohol a

---

[3] Article on this in *Evening Post, 2/8/06*
[4] The detail here is based on the Home Office publication, *Prospects. Bristol Female Project, Snowdon Rd. Questions and answers* (26/08/2005) Home Office

day from off sales and supermarkets. When you get to that stage, pubs are more than double the price for alcohol, and the alcoholic content subsumes the drinker over any taste or fun had getting drunk. Even with his habit, it is hard for everyone to be able to afford £175 a week for alcohol or £350 on heroin. The time of imbibing and recovery takes more hours a day than would fit with routines of occupation and domesticity on the outside.

The houses, one for men and one for women, opened amid a storm of Nimby protest as local residents objected to concentrations of people of this kind being in their neighbourhood. People don't want others that have suffered and been forced to fight in unacceptable ways to survive. The fear of a group of people concentrated together who have committed crime in the past, irrational because these people would be in more precarious a position and living in the same area anyway, Fishponds being no high class neighbourhood.

Drug treatment programmes save £1.10 for every £1 spent on them[5]. Prospects is in its infancy, being a first statutory sector step to take drugs offenders out of the prison system in this way. From the author's standpoint, halfway housing on the way from mental hospital is a welcome chance for one to rehabilitate from one situation to the more dangerous and stressful "Real World".

---

[5] See interview with Aileen Edwards at the end of this chapter.

For better or worse, people are confined in mental hospital against their will, there is a routine, rules, and a culture of the confined in both, why not apply these lessons to the prison system as well?

Andrew would experience supported housing after being confined in the secure mental health system. Time now to rejoin Andrew where he got housed by the council after another spell in prison…

Things changed for the better when I got housed. I was released on the Friday, there were a couple of parties to go to so I had somewhere to crash. At some point that weekend I got a black eye, no idea how because I was so drunk. On the Monday I went to see my probation officer. My mail was redirected there and in that was an offer of a flat from the council! Went down, looked at it and took it. I was on the dole but needed some money so took a cash in hand job window cleaning. One of the addresses we done, the garage was open and I saw a three piece suite. I offered the woman some money for it and got the suite. Somewhere to sleep! She was also throwing out a washing machine. I looked at it and the pump was leaking, she gave it me and I fitted a new pump. Got given an old gas cooker by a mate… in this way I gathered the basics for living in my own home.

Anyway my mate Mike and I noticed two girls moving into a flat nearby. We helped them move in and they invited us to dinner. My turn next, cooked a chicken dinner for the 4 of us, and Mike got together with one of them. They got married within weeks, funny as we'd agreed not to get involved in anything on our doorstep! While they were infatuated, Karen and I got together. She fell pregnant. After the new arrival there was a damp patch on the wall around one of the electrical sockets. We told the council but they ignored us, so we got the local press in to take photos and run a story on it. Still nothing was done so we got the fire brigade in and they said the flat was dangerous to live in. The council moved us into a 3 bed semi with a garden. Kaz fell pregnant again and we had our second child.

She and I had a deal, happy me smoking dope but she didn't like my drinking. I'd disappear for a few days to get pissed, and come home when the money ran out. I was allowed to smoke cannabis in the house, so stoned I was there with our friends. People would come round to play on the Sega Mega Drive for a few hours, others would come to play cards, and we had a dinner party circuit. Thinking back, I should have shared the responsibilities of running the house with her. Paid all the bills, made sure we had money for all the things we needed, got maintenance done. It all got a bit much for me, I guess that's one of the reasons I would snap when I eventually did.

One night I came in and lost the plot – started smashing the decorations up with a hammer. Kaz came down and calmed me down. She went to bed, but I stayed up, sure that someone was going to harm the family. The telly seemed to be talking *about me. Hard to explain… It was all of a sudden too. One moment I was fine and the next I was in this parallel universe where people were after me. Completely freaked out. Kaz took the kids out in the morning. I was so paranoid I got tooled up with a load of kitchen knives. The problems were in the house so I had to get out, just outside – anywhere but there. I ran out the garden, jumped over the wall and started walking the streets... Someone jumped up really quickly behind me on a bus so I slashed out, injuring but not killing him. I ran off and slowed down a bit. I was walking the streets again and someone ran up behind me so I stabbed him – this time I pierced his heart.*

I got picked up by the police later that day. I admitted it, they told me to empty out my pockets and a load of knives fell out…

How does it feel to experience a different reality to what most consider normal? From the author's perspective, it actually feels normal insofar as there is no apparent difference between normality and the experiences of this illness. "Real" and "unreal" are identical to perceive. Hunter S Thompson, who will be dealt with in the chapter *A Mad World*, described a mescaline trip and used the same words to describe hundreds of bats flying over his car outside Las Vegas as the casual observer would outside a bat cave at dusk. Distinguishing what is real and what is not is key. Having a stomach full of chemicals tells you that this is not real. But imagine you had not taken enough acid to burn through Woodstock and things suddenly changed?

What follows is an account of my own experiences of paranoid schizophrenia. A leap of imagination is needed here. In order to get across the strange, disjointed experience of schizophrenia, I have written my story as told by a listener to a radio station that I listen to, and talk to...

"There's this bloke who talks over the music. Swears a lot too, and brings up issues that children will ask their mothers about... "Mummy, what does he mean when he says truckers ass fuck their mothers?" Try explaining THAT to a 7 year old!

When the film The Truman Show *came out, everyone thought Rich would be let out like Truman was at the end of the film – the film being about a man who is brought up on a TV set without knowing he was the star of a prime time show. I thought he'd be told by the producers, or arrested for radio piracy. No one did anything, telling the real life Truman about his being permanently on air. He knew something was wrong and kept on asking them to help him out. When he was diagnosed with mental illness, I thought it was some way of bringing it to an end. No.*

The DJ's aren't allowed to talk back to him directly so they talk to him indirectly. Recently, Russell Brand let him know his view of him by playing

Suicide is Painless *by the Manic Street Preachers on BBC 6Music. Served the guy right, hates Brand and had been playing free jazz over the guy's output for the last hour! Some of the DJ's like him. Must be fun someone randomly talking back to you when you're in the studio playing records and doing your skits. Truly, interactive radio, way better than text messages telling them what the listeners think of the new track by The Editors! Rich says outright "Indy clones" or occasionally some sort of compliment. They do get annoyed with him though. The Russell Brand incident was classic. He can start to rant if the DJ's tell him to get lost, which rather defeats the objective of getting him to shut up.*

He's been on air since about 1996. At about the same time, the fly on the wall documentary was coming of age so this was nothing unusual. Rather than some transsexual prostitute walking the streets of Paddington and showing off to the camera, this was a real man making his way through the world. You could hear him puzzled a bit when DJ's started talking back to him. We thought it was a joke or something, but none of the press took it up. Listening to a guy finishing his degree and going through the trials and tribulations of life without really knowing he was doing it. He talks about his life and commentates on politics. I wish I had the ability to tell politicians "you're wrong", must be so empowering. The ultimate in Blair's "stakeholder - led society", the people fronting their leaders as opposed to some stuffed shirt columnist in the Times. *Everyone else gets one chance every 5 years but Rich exercises his democratic right every time he chooses!*

The authorities had him diagnosed with schizophrenia. He'd been on air for 3 years when it happened. Never went quiet though, no matter what drugs they put him on. So doped up on that shit, he slept 16 hours a day and complained he could have 3 hours between thinking anything. You'd've thought MI5 or someone would want to find out more? Get spies to do it or something! They tried to lock him away instead. Hates the Government, and always comes up with different ideas for policy. When the IRA bombed Omagh he knew the history of the Troubles and told them to stop, and how to stop it. Some think him responsible for the peace process, uniting people against violence.

But he's angry all the same. He was a leader of the anti-globalisation movement and told them to meet at Parliament Square for a protest and plant trees there while a group of them would storm the House of Commons and throw out the politicians. A revolution! The authorities had him diagnosed the day before – whack. Just like the Soviet Union, throwing enemies of the State in the loony bin."

+++++++++++++

So the listener explains that I live in *The Truman Show*. Here is how it feels to be "Truman" and aware that something just ain't right. I recount the parallel reality…

"I talk and to the TV and radio. The DJ's communicate back. Subtly – they make inferences in their speech and in the tracks they play;

I say "Russell Brand is a media whore who shags sluts"

He replies by playing Suicide is painless *by Manic Street Preachers or another track of poignant message. By this interpretation on my part and apparent listening on the DJ's part, relationships were born years ago and have been fostered.*

I have tried to communicate with them directly. To my understanding they want me to talk about issues they want, talking to them about the music they play or entering competitions. I can't do that, have never done that because I am the one who has been diagnosed by the state health service as being of a dangerous and life threatening illness, they want me to speak to them on their terms?! Before diagnosis I was phoning them every night and emailing from internet cafes. Doing this, to get this thing out in the open and leave it behind, to accept that I can be heard when I talk in front of a radio. They refuse to talk to me about this issue – by phone, email or anything. Instead, a stalking pattern emerges as I tell them to talk to me on the phone or by email and they do not. Personally, if I wanted to stalk someone I'd stalk real celebrity like George Monbiot, not some airhead DJ. All I wanted to do was get this thing cleared up. Uri

GIVING VOICE TO THE INNER SCREAM

Gellar has cutlery he can't bend – get me a stereo that doesn't talk back!

The last book I read was Bob Dylan's Chronicles, Volume 1. *Half the Radio One DJs don't know who he is! They make me feel like a misfit because I am interested in people who've lived a life. One of them plugged Wayne Rooney's book the other week. A "good read". A 19 year old's autobiography must be riveting, can just see the single reference to sex in the massage parlour he went to pop his cherry because the England team were taking the piss out of him for being a virgin. Give me a break!*

If the radio thing were real then I have been a thorn in the government's side. I am the only person on BBC output with a commentary column. The job of the 4th Estate (as the media is known) is as counterweight to the 1st (Monarchy), 2nd (Legislature) and 3rd (Judiciary) - to criticise. Other broadcasters criticise by questioning, Jeremy Paxman and John Snow being kings among broadcast journalists. I am not constrained by broadcasting law (which discourages opinion in news) and criticise with opinion, Paxman and Snow not being allowed.

So I live two lives. I have the definite life, where I am campaigning against the stigma of mental illness in society. I have an apparent life where I am a columnist on the radio. I wish I knew from staff at the BBC if this was real and not just psychiatrists saying otherwise because I could keep it or lose it. Psyches hear this story all the time, knowing that makes them unreliable. They just say "take my word for it – we know it's a brain malfunction". I am an intelligent person with an inquisitive mind, you have got to prove me wrong and not treat me like some psychotic inebriate[6]. I had a good contact at BBC Plymouth. A producer who worked with me when I was on placement there. The relationship broke down when I asked her to help me get to the bottom of the illness. I couldn't explain eloquently what I perceived, so got angry and frustrated with her, she getting confused and scared of me as I insisted she use her contacts in BBC national radio to find out if I am nuts or not. For a broadcast journalist, a producer at the BBC as a friend is a key ally in getting your career off the ground… until you stuff it by acting crazy with her.

Now I am worried that the neighbours have been annoyed to the point that they have complained and that the tenancy for this flat, due for renewal in a month's time, will not be renewed. Tonight I told the radio I don't want to be heard every time I scratch my bollocks. The DJ did a link there and then about the bin men at the festival she was at, a clear hint that my going was the trash being taken out. But it will communicate with me again,

---

[6] "Psychiatric mystification is a powerful influence in the maintenance of people's oppression" **Innovative Psychotherapies** by R. Corsini.

and I with it. Neighbours will be annoyed - I just hope the same ones as this time..."

++++++++++++++++++++++

In many ways Andrew was lucky in meeting a writer who had exactly the same symptoms as he did. Either that or he listens to me on the radio! Other symptoms include the classic "invisible people talking to you" (voices), but may include touch and visual hallucinations such as snakes crawling over your body. This list is not exhaustive. What causes them? With medicine at an apparent height of its powers, there must be an understanding of the biology of the illness?

No. The brain is the least understood organ of the body. Its function can only be studied with the brain functioning. One can see what a liver does by removing it, dissecting and running tests on it to see which chemicals it produces. One can then look at other parts of the body to disseminate where those chemicals go, and from there, what those chemicals do. The body from which the liver comes may be dead, yet one can deduce the function of the liver as the body was when it was alive.

The brain is an organ that manages the entire body. If it is dead and cannot move an arm, one cannot see what part fires to move the arm. In the 20th Century, medicine became advanced enough to operate on the brain with the patient conscious – so surgeons could apply electrodes to parts of the brain to see what part did what. Establishing motor function and other simple processes that they could trigger from the surface of the brain. To complex issues such as conscious processes of abstract thought and behaviour – what are the neuro-chemical processes while the patient is engaging in play and sex with a lover? Couldn't remove the top of the skull and attach electrodes, a major turnoff having sex with someone with the skull half removed, and pillow talk would be almost impossible. What are the processes involved in social interaction of any kind? What differs between normal social processes and the disrupted processes of the mind regarded as being mentally ill?

What of the biology of schizophrenia? I spoke to Dr Stanley Zammit, lecturer of Psychological Medicine at Cardiff and Bristol Universities.

The biological illness.

Psychosis as a biological entity can be seen as increased dopamine levels in the mesolimbic cortex of the brain with decreased levels in the prefrontal cortex. There also seems to be less glutamate in the psychotic's brain. This can be seen when one induces psychosis in human brains in clinical trials by giving drugs like THC, the active ingredient of cannabis, intravenously. The psychotic's brain is on average smaller than one of sound mind, and the ventricles are spaced farther apart.

Those are the facts. Here is where the mud enters the water. The brain that does not show symptoms of psychosis may have the same electrochemical and physical attributes as the brain that does. The appearance of biological symptoms are trends rather than measurable biological events, no specific centre being in the brain to explain this where this happens such as a brain cancer.

1000 brains. Statistically 10 will have psychosis. 7 may have brain structure and chemistry that are different to the brains of "sound mind". 3 "sound minds" of the 1000 may have close similarities with those 7! There is no biological measure for psychosis. No blood test, no brain smears available. There are links between activity in the patient's mind and chemistry but so far the chemistry and neural activity measures are too general. It is like the scenario where the Italian man is on average 5 ft 10 and the British man is on average 5 ft 11. This does not mean a 5 ft 10 is Italian and the 5 ft 11 is British!

Drug induced psychosis

Cannabis can definitely cause psychosis, and is used to induce it for study of the psychotic brain. However the psychosis measured disappears within hours or days of the dose being given. The evidence that it causes long term harm (schizophrenia for instance) is circumstantial only. There is no scientific evidence to show that cannabis can cause psychosis except over the period that it is physically in the brain.

There is another disease that we can only link circumstantially to the misuse of drugs – heart disease and smoking. There are no permanent, biologically measurable changes in the heart caused by nicotine or whatever other nasties get in the blood through the smoke. The lifestyle of the heart patient and the smoker will have similarities. Regardless of whether he smokes he may be overweight, get little exercise and have a poor diet, all of which also contribute to heart disease. To another illness, an author of several antismoking books who had quit smoking 23 years before was diagnosed with lung cancer. Was it smoking? Or was he going to get it anyway? The dope smoker will lead a similar lifestyle to the man who does not smoke dope and will get psychosis anyway. But there are people who lead the same lifestyle who will not get psychosis!

Scientific observation of psychosis

The neurobiological science of schizophrenia is maybe 20 years old, of which the best science has been done since 2000. This has come about with the use of CAT, MRI and PET scans in research. These can show the chemistry and neural activity in the brains of the research subject.

You cannot give a rat psychosis. There is no way of measuring its conscious brain activity. If a man can say the radio is talking to him specifically, what would a rat with psychosis say?

GIVING VOICE TO THE INNER SCREAM

[Hunter A Thompson describes a mescaline trip of hundreds of cats flying over the rat run…]

You can give a rat lung cancer. You can test how the disease progresses from there and you can kill the rat to look at its lungs. You can talk to the human about the radio talking to him specifically, but you cannot kill the human to look at his brain activity. Medical ethics, and just think of the press coverage![7] Scanning has enabled some inroads into this situation – one can now see what is going on without taking off part of their skull or killing them.

There are symptoms of schizophrenia that may be treated. Delusions are most common [such as the radio thing described above]. The sufferer may hallucinate, whether hearing voices, feeling things on the skin, even tasting things. They may have broken up thought patterns and show incoherence in speech. Poor motivation, he might not go to the supermarket to buy his food for the week and starve instead. "Flattened affect" is a symptom where the sufferer has difficulty feeling emotions.

Medication

Two people of schizoid condition may suffer from totally different symptoms yet may be on the same

---

[7] Read Andrew Scull's *A most solitary of afflictions* pp 226 – 228 for an insight into phrenology, a Victorian science of dead patients' skulls being measured for difference from sane people. It was discredited, no doubt in part because of the press…

dose of the same medication. Medication is traditionally a large part of the stigma of mental illness. The so called "typical antipsychotics" such as haloperidol and Stelazine have some side effects that are quite debilitating and obvious. They might include muscle tremors, the production of too much saliva so that the patient drools, and heavy sedation. These drugs have been used since the 1950's and do reduce the symptoms of schizophrenia, to the same extent that the newer drugs do. The drugs have the knock on effect of the stereotypical medicated patient that is lampooned in society. Electroconvulsive therapy (ECT), zapping the brain in the most feared of psychiatric treatments, is effective too. This is now not socially acceptable, though unlike older radical treatments such as insulin therapy, it works. It is of such stigma and fear that it is rarely used.

There are new drugs on the market that have been in use for the last 20 or so years. These are known as "atypical antipsychotics". They do not have the same ugly side effects as the typicals, but do cause others. The patient may gain weight and sleep more for instance. The National Institute for Clinical Excellence (NICE) has directed that in most cases the patient should be put on these more expensive medicines rather than the cheaper, older ones because the side effects are less severe for the recipient[8]. Bluntly the twitching

---

[8] NICE explanation of antipsychotic policy
http://www.nice.nhs.uk/page.aspx?o=CG001

drooly will be stared at in the street whereas the overweight man won't!

Summary

As far as is known, mental illness is primarily a software fault rather than a hardware fault. We cannot look at Andrew's life as he was living it and say "you're going to get schizophrenia if you continue". His grandmother was a case in point, a heavy smoker until she died of natural causes. The smoking should have given her cancer or heart disease if the doctors knew that smoking kills for certain – it doesn't. He had a traumatic life. But equally people without trauma in their lives are diagnosed with psychosis. It has been shown that trauma in the womb can lead to schizophrenia. So the man who went without recreational drugs, led a sheltered childhood, could still be diagnosed with the illness because his Mum might have been to heavy metal concerts while she was pregnant and he as a foetus didn't like the moshing in the mosh pit! Schizophrenia is a disease of the mind that can be controlled biologically. We cannot measure the symptoms biologically, and two people may have completely different symptoms in the mind but have the same diagnosis. We do not know exactly what the drugs do but they seem to work!

Understanding is key to judgement. Mental illness has not been understood in the hundreds of years it has been treated, and lampooned in society as a result. The lack of medical understanding and no rationale in society lends to fear and thus the stigma. Zammit states that no biomedical explanation has yet tackled the stigma. The media, the surest litmus of society and catalyst of society's views, is next on this hit parade of misunderstanding.

Asian people suffer from stigmatisation in Western society because they have the same appearance as people who fly planes into skyscrapers. People who practice Islam at a mosque are seen as potentially subversive because some mullahs suggest that violence is the way to defend Islam against the corrupting influences of Western Christendom. The media reports on the unusual and the feared. A mullah who says "live and let live" to the mosque is less likely to be seen on TV, except in times of crisis, than the hook handed bugger who says Christendom is evil and needs a good drubbing! After one of the crises, that the peaceful mullah would appear on TV calling for understanding, in September 2001, I saw a family in Afghan dress, including a woman in a burkha. These people, in dress, were the enemy and a threat to the civilisation in which I lived. 9/11 was a media event to tell the world that the nutters wanted a fight.

The media is similarly responsible for the bulk of the stigma of mental illness[9]. Nothing like the race and religion laws prevent people from calling me a loony or the press from hounding a psychiatric

---

[9] Greg Philo (1995) "Media and mental distress" amongst *many* other publications

patient from his job at John Lewis in Bristol because of a crime he committed 10 years ago. From personal experience the media does not only attack the vulnerable outside its ivory towers but those inside. CNN's London bureau recently sacked someone for having depression[10] and a newspaper is facing an Employment Tribunal over allegations it made, which were used at the time to sack a senior reporter who has mental illness[11].

For someone like myself writing this, being of an oppressed minority that even the BBC sees fit to brand as a type of person demarcated by the illness I suffer, I lead a life of regular and unregulated disdain by the uninformed, foul mouthed hounds of the media. The term "gutter press" springs to mind but must include every UK media outlet in this particular net. Andrew *is* the bogeyman the press refers to each time it slanders me and mine. To some extent because of the wrongs he committed, he deserves an element of disdain because what he did was morally and ethically against the most basic standards we keep as mankind. But this man has been found by the courts to not be responsible for his actions.

One has newspaper clippings about the events that cannot be printed in the interests of Andrew's anonymity. The conclusion drawn is that, in writing a good story the media elicited fear in the public

---

[10] The Journalist (August 2006) National Union of Journalists
[11] She has recently been moved to a secure psychiatric unit as a result.

about mental illness. The immediate secondary victims were Andrew's young family. His kids were too young to go to school and get it for his actions but Kaz suffered for association with a man of diseased mind. The media coverage was such that Andrew's children have had their names changed so when they did attend school, school gate tittle tattle did not pre-empt bullying. There were a multitude of tertiary victims of this crime. Two people were stabbed by a loony before the media started frothing at the mouth and stabbed 1% of the entire population in the back with hysterical press coverage about how dangerous "schizophrenics" are. (1% of humanity has schizophrenia). The cliché that nothing should get in the way of a good story makes the bulk of people with similar neurobiological events a feared segment of society.

Andrew will never get away from the label because of the Home Office's restrictions on his liberty. I will never get away from this label either – because I have chosen to stand on the rooftops crying out that I have this illness and that you are wrong in stigmatising me. The difference between Andrew and I is that he is labelled of compunction, I of volition.

The next section takes on Andrew's detention and recovery. It is interesting that I had to pause the final interview three times to speak to my father. The issue with Dad was over a damaged car he had given me and then got angry with me during its MOT, which it would fail catastrophically. I asked Andrew who the nut in the room was. He laughed. Andrew takes up the story from his arrest.

I got picked up by the police later that day. I admitted it, they told me to empty out my pockets and a load of knives fell out.

Something funny happened at that point. I only have flashes of memory for about 3 months. I was at a committal at a Magistrates Court. I was put on remand in prison. I smashed up the cell, chucking the mattress out the window and ripping the toilet and sink off the wall, I was sitting in an inch of water at the end of that. Basically I was arrested, put in a cell, seen by a doctor, then a psychiatrist, and put in the hospital wing. While I was there I was processed through the Court system, where I was found unfit to stand trial. The screws told me I was moving and took me to Rampton.

Once there I was stripped, showered, and given a Bic razor to shave off my full beard, that bit took about 2 hours. I was put on the Admissions Ward where I punched someone for winding me up. In the Admissions Ward, you're there for assessment and the staff figure out what treatment to put you on. The psychiatrist decided I was mad because sat outside I like to give shapes to clouds ("that looks like a plane, that a house"). The psychologist laughed, saying that if I was mad because of that, he must be too since he did the same thing! The psychologist got more out of you because they knew how, the psychiatrist was just concerned about what pills to put you on. At that point, I didn't understand mental illness. It took me 10 years to get to grips with it.

Though I committed the crime, I was reacting to things that my brain told me that weren't true. My brain lied to me and I reacted to its lies by attacking people that the brain told me were going to attack me.

You're in there for as long as it takes to get well. Some in for psychiatric assessment, were there for as little as 28 days, and were sent back to the prison system because the psychiatrists thought them fit to stand trial. I was there for about 9 years for treatment. People used to debate whether Rampton was a prison hospital or a psychiatric unit. Here's the difference. Prison hospital, you're locked in your cell most of the time and in Special Hospital you're on the ward, mixing with the others. Doing bird, I was let out my cell twice, and that was for a bath, even my food given me through a hatch. You said that you imagined that prison hospital is a dormitory (like in the comedy, Porridge*) but the reality is that many people are mentally ill in that wing and clash with each other so in most cases they're put in cells.*

After a time I was moved on to an intermediate ward. The sexes were segregated but I saw women when I was waiting to see the doctor or whatever. It's interesting that there were some really nice looking women there with rubbery skin from all the self harming they done. I guess when men get angry they lash out, women harm themselves.

I got a job making pottery. Paid £3 a session, which bought my fags. When I started, there was a metal working and a tailoring shop but these closed down. What that meant was that there was nothing to do most of the time. Horticulture was an escape that also bought me fags! We had everything from potatoes to tomatoes. We also kept chickens and ducks for eggs, which were sold to service users. [Asked if kept for meat, no!] The daily routine was simple. We got up, had breakfast, and did the horticulture from about 9.30 to lunch. In the afternoons we had nothing to do so played pool, watched telly and read. With pool, we had to get the staff to sign the pool cues out so we could play - otherwise someone might get hit with it. We weren't allowed lighters so there was a machine on the wall where you pressed a button and a bit would glow red. To combat the boredom, some of us got together and got our own greenhouse and looked after that.

Even though we had keys to our rooms, rooms you could lock from the inside, security was tight. After intermediate I was moved to a villa. These were large houses with 20 bedrooms or so but you were allowed to walk in the grounds. We were given security passes and could wander outside. Outside the villa area was a huge ditch, beyond that, a 15 metre high fence and a road for security to drive down and on the other side of that, another fence. One time we got a hose for our polytunnel. I was having a casual chat with the security guy and said we had the hose and were waiting for the tap to attach it to. He said he'd be back later, came and took the hose away. If you can imagine two 45 ft fences, a road and a ditch, how were we meant to throw the end of the hose over all that?

In prison you can get almost anything you want, drink or drugs are no problem. It's much harder to get stuff in hospital. If you're really lucky you can get a bit of dope but what's the point? You're there to get well and cannabis doesn't let you. You get paranoid again and that kicks off psychosis. In theory they could have kept me in for the rest of my life so I made the decision to never drink again. For instance, they sold Kaliber in there – couldn't see the point in drinking it as it would just give me the taste for booze. When I was in Fromeside, I could have gone to the pub on the corner. My decision was that alcohol takes away your control of your life so the simple answer is not to drink. Imagine if I'd been drinking one night and blacked out? I'd shit meself when I came to! Alcoholics Anonymous wouldn't work for me. My understanding about drink is that you have to make the decision for yourself and it's not others to make that decision for you. I couldn't quit drink because others want me to.

I do want the Home Office to allow me to go to the pub. I don't want to drink there – I just want to be recognised as a local, a regular. I want to meet people and be accepted. There's my License and my health, I'm too old to do all that again.

My parents are getting on a bit and I didn't want to go back to Essex. Sister lives in Bristol so I asked the authorities whether I could be sent here. For my Mum and Step Dad to travel one weekend down to Bristol and then another, to say Birmingham, would be a real challenge for them so having both kids in one place would make it simpler. The powers that be agreed. I did 9 years in Rampton and about two in Fromeside, Bristol. This is what they call a "regional secure unit", half way between the special hospital and the normal mental hospital ward. You've met me here in Bristol half way house. I moved there under Home Office License.

Looking to the future I have the perfect scenario for you. I get up, go to work, go to the pub for a couple of hours, and home to fuck the girlfriend. That would be all my hopes in life in one day. Problems are a few things. Firstly there's the issue of needing one day a week to see my professionals. The Home Office needs a report on my well being every three months, so I need to see my professionals to send in that report. What employer's going to take me on 4 days a week? Social Work is a 9 – 5 job, and they aren't going to do overtime. Given my stay in mental hospital for as long as I have, what employer would have me? The stigma of mental illness is so strong that I see getting any job as an achievement… Let's face it, I have to say that I have done Life because of my crime on my application form. From what I understand it is hard enough if you only spent 6 months in hospital nowadays, let alone 10 years.

Finally, my kids've changed their names. The case was getting a lot of publicity and they were getting to school age. The wife didn't want people to recognise her name and to gossip. Imagine parents finding out and then the kids - you know what kids are like, they'd bully them. Kaz also decided to not allow me to see them again. It hurts, that is the worst bit of the punishment I have had, but at the end of the day the kids' safety is paramount. If they don't know their Dad for that to be the case, then it's better for them.

Between 30 and 50% of the single person homeless population have mental health problems[12]. In the 1980's an organisation came together in Bristol called Second Step. This voluntary sector organisation provides housing for people with psychiatric history or drug and alcohol problems. Several exist locally; North Britain and Carr Gomm being another two.

Andrew's house had all mod cons; a shower room as well as a bathroom, a garden and a fully equipped kitchen. The living room became equipped with a 28 inch widescreen TV and a sound system due to four solvent bachelors living there! The regime is for each service user to

---

[12] Centrepoint (2006) Making the link between mental health and youth homelessness, a pan – London study Mental Health Foundation

receive about 3 hours of support a week, whether talking therapy or basic things like taking them shopping at the supermarket or cleaning their rooms. The staff would be there generally two afternoons a week. It is a family house that in most ways would resemble that of any other in the street except that four men who lived there were on state benefits and they were visited during office hours by young to middle aged women... Though not for the services most men would want!

Supporting People is dealt with in the next chapter. It is a national scheme that funds society's most vulnerable, from old people to the blind, that require tenancy and basic living support. What is left to be said is how the supported housing system works in Bristol. I interviewed Aileen Edwards, the Director of Second Step.

The organisation was set up in 1987 with a cluster of bed-sits in Cotham in Bristol. Initially run by volunteers and Community Psychiatric Nurses, its aim was to prevent psychiatric service users from becoming homeless. Over the years it has become an accepted method of housing people in the city. What Second Step did was arrange this in the form of family sized (3-5 people) units. It was a struggle at first, up to then most housing of this type was of the hostel or hospital variety. In these forms, supported housing has been in existence as long as psychiatric patients have been treated. We now run 20 properties and are still growing, providing support for nearly 1000 people.

There are no statistics to measure the success of our projects. No way has been developed as yet[13], though we do know that about 75% of our clients are seen to have moved out in what we call a positive way – not hospital for instance. Another statistic is that for every £1 spent on drug rehabilitation, £1.10 is saved by the government; a 10% saving on a UK wide basis is a lot of money!

About ¾ of our funding is from the Government scheme Supporting People. This money is for the support of people in need, paying for the care whilst the Council pays the rent in the way it would for most disabled people. Since being imposed in 2003 there has not been an inflationary increase in the fund as would be the case for the NHS. This means we are constantly having to trim our margins to provide the same level of support for the people we serve[14]. The government has changed our sector's name from the Voluntary Sector to the Third Sector, showing that it has long term aims for us in mind. I hope that one day that Second Step and the other organisations in Bristol may provide a place for service users instead of hospital.

---

[13] A system is being worked out now for government statistics

[14] Author's note - As this is written there has been news that Supporting People is getting a decrease in funding because of government faddism and bureaucracy. Read the next chapter for a greater insight...

GIVING VOICE TO THE INNER SCREAM

This last point that Aileen raised is worth looking at. With the trends for the care in the community model now leaving the mental health world and hospital inpatient care being provided for only the most acute of any illness, this is again happening to a much greater extent in the mental health world. The provision of care outside is actually more intensive in some ways than that provided on an acute ward; the author was in for 6 weeks and only saw my key worker there once. There for a compulsory alcohol detox, other than being prevented from leaving the building, I was all but ignored. In the community, I had the support at home, was being seen by a Community Psychiatric Nurse for one hour a week's Cognitive Behavioural Therapy, monthly interviews with my psychiatrist, was attending a Clifton NHS alcohol detox day centre (group and one to one therapy), as well as being able to use the day hospital in Redland, you'll see my workload as an outpatient far more intensive than that found in inpatient care!

Andrew has moved on now. I last interviewed him at his Bristol supported housing. We agreed that he be given anonymity because of the press that may want to hunt him down and expose him for the crime of being mentally ill. Part of that agreement is that I don't know where he moved to.

Safety Net

As described in the previous chapter, supported housing is a system for getting people of a variety of backgrounds to reacquaint with and rejoin society. The system in place can be for the physically disabled, the elderly, homeless people and most importantly for me in my recovery, the mentally ill.

Though not always specific to mental health and the stigma associated with it, this chapter looks at the effects of government foot dragging amidst the two pressures of doing the right thing and bean counting in the Treasury. The public's public eye is the media, and this is a case of a Meerkat making its call for the gang to react – "I see you Gordon and Tony, let's not strike too soon."

The mentally ill are often stigmatised as "weak" and incapable of dealing with society in the normal way. By providing that support to go to the shops with underpants under your trousers (and not over, as one pop song suggested) and to get the strength to get a job and not "sponge", supported accommodation provides the ability for vulnerable groups to participate in society with little notice, and thrive in that society among the many mores and conventions it has.

In short, supported accommodation fights the stigma in its own right, by enabling people to rise above the charge of departing from society's systems. Why report on it? The government, which set out to provide it with sound footing in *Supporting People*, is gently cutting its funding. Shaving for the moment, we shall see if the shave becomes a visit to the barbers rather than the morning ablutions of late.

In 1999 I moved into supported housing. My Social Worker thought this a place for me to recuperate more effectively within than that of my tiny bed-sit up the road in Redland. My "supported house" was a shared house for five male psychiatric patients, a shared house with a support worker who worked into the property. Her job was to ensure that there was harmony among the residents, and individually, to help us find our feet again in society.

This last job was the original intent for Second Step when it was started in 1987[15], with three properties in the Bristol area. The bills are paid; electricity, gas and TV License are covered in the rent that was paid by Housing Benefit. The support was given with the intent that people; who might have been institutionalised for some time, could shop for themselves, make new friends; and find their way in the world.

Up to about 2002, Housing Benefit paid the bulk of the costs associated with living in such a property. In 2002 a new scheme was mooted, *Supporting People (SP)*, which would provide for all the support needs associated with supported living in

---

[15] A brief history is in the previous chapter

the UK other than rent, which would be covered with Housing Benefit.

Transitional Housing Benefit (THB) was created in the run up to *SP* being launched in April 2003. Local Authorities were told to go ahead and provide the support needs of their clients, and a number of councils in the UK took this with both hands, setting up schemes that covered a range of support needs; the homeless, ex drug users, psychiatric patients, and the physically disabled figuring large among this group. This was meant to give the government some idea as to how big the supported housing costs would be in the UK. The response, though mixed between authorities overall, came as a shock to the Treasury. *Supporting People* was thought to eventually cost under £1 billion; it came to nearly £2 billion!

On the so-called SP Day, 1 April 2003, mental health supported housing attained £250 million[16] of a £1.8 billion total pot for vulnerable people to be supported in their tenancies in England. On publication of the Robson Rhodes LLP Report in January 2004, it became apparent that there was a wild variation in the unit cost of providing that support to people across the nation. Through this chapter, I will look at the reasons that funding was frozen at 2003 levels and is decreed that it should be more efficiently distributed.

---

[16] Robson Rhodes LLP Report 2004

GIVING VOICE TO THE INNER SCREAM

Over the succeeding years, supported housing providers have faced a classic Treasury response, a funding freeze. With inflation at or about 3% for the last three years, there has been an effective cut in funding of 3% per year in relation to inflation. In 2007 the scheme faces a cut by the government.

Having had five years of support, and a space of five years in which to recover and recuperate from the rigours of mental illness, I look back to my time in Second Step's support with warmth. To a time where I was not concerned with having to earn my crust to pay for everything while my brain was wired the wrong way, and a chance to reflect and change direction in life at my own pace. So I was shocked when I heard that in Bristol, the 5000 people receiving support through *SP* in Bristol could face a 30% cut in funding. Why? Who's responsible? What will be the repercussions?

I went to speak to a man who set up on his own with Supporting People, to look after his 30 year old son with a dual diagnosis of cerebral palsy and psychosis. John Wallace and wife Cathy had to support their son; a job that took 60 hours a week, before they achieved independent living for Ian. They're now contracted to provide 25 hours of support a week as Ian forges forward toward a life of almost total independence despite his disabling conditions.

"Traditionally the young are brought up in the family to age 16 or shortly after, and they fly the

nest. My daughter followed this line, and is a friendly face now and again in my house, I am the same at hers. We help each other out as families do, eventually she may spend more time looking after my needs than I her. Many kids now go to university and get financial backing from their parents, but even so this is the chick fledging and learning to live on their own with some input from the parents.

In my son's case, when he was 26 I was spending 60 hours a week looking after him. This is not the level of support a 26 year old should need, and frankly I am too old to do this for the rest of his life! In 2002 I discovered that I could get the State to provide support for Ian. Basically the Housing Benefit rules were that I could put him up in his own flat and be funded to look after him.

Ian is not wheelchair bound and is quite active. Being able to walk and get around is something he is lucky with, many with cerebral palsy don't have that luxury. However he developed psychosis in his early 20's which made him need as much support as perhaps he'd need if he was severely disabled by CP. With his psychosis he was difficult to have around in the house. Cabin fever, meaning an adult son in the home with his parents with all the issues of living together, and psychosis does not contribute to a wonderful family nest.

Moving him into his own flat quickly dealt with the cabin fever, and dealing with him was made that much easier. Being able to get people in to provide housing support needs gave a variety of faces to Ian's life, and that is what he badly needed - a life. With a "life" you have a variety of people around you and you do different things. Prior to this he would be in my house for days, weeks on end, rattling around and fighting with me and his mother Cathy.

In 2003 Housing Benefit was scheduled to change to a nationally run scheme, Supporting People (SP) which is a centrally funded (but locally administered) system of grants to provide housing support for the disabled and vulnerable groups in society. Transitional Housing Benefit (THB) was designed in 2002 to lead up to what was called "SP Day" on the 1st April 2003.

THB was an unlimited pot of money for support in the community. It was done to get a handle on what money would be required for the Supporting People pot. Run by the Office of the Deputy Prime Minister, it was seen as a way to make Housing Benefit an equitable benefit, provided to everyone in need of rent payments from the State and covering only rent. Importantly SP was a pot of cash for support. Thus two men living in rooms in shared housing, rent £75 a week, would get the £70 a week HB under SP. The man in supported housing would originally get say £200 a week to cover his support needs whilst the man without support needs would get the same £70 a week. The man without would rightly question this originally, perhaps asking whether he might live in a decent sized flat in a good area for the same price?

But to me this meant getting Ian into a setting in which a man in his late 20's should be in; independently and with reference to his parents, not being parented by them. I fought hard for this and became the UK's only single client recipient of Supporting People. As it turned out the door that I got through to receive this closed behind me, making it impossible for other parents in my situation to get the grant.

The barriers that came down were of classic bureaucratese, funding. Only those with the support provision and secure tenure of occupancy on SP Day would get SP. Under THB we had bought him a flat (the costs for which came out of our life savings) and we set up the monitoring system required. Some funding has become available since, but to my knowledge no other family in the UK has managed to get it.

On the 1st April 2003, THB became SP. A grand day for governance, but the Treasury was not happy; the initial estimate was £700 million and with all the support given nationally it came to something like £1.8 billion!

The money from SP is for "support" which is differentiated from "care". With Ian he cannot use his hands very well. Thus he needs to be washed and helped to cook his dinner, as well as paying his rent on time and looking after his Direct

Payments to his care team. Support amounts to teaching him how to cook, ensuring that he cleans his flat so it is a safe place in which to live, making sure he pays his carers. Care amounts to helping him wash, physiotherapy... right up to neurosurgery.

Supporting People ring fences the stuff I do for my son as a professional and what I do as his Dad. I am a professional housing supporter now, as well as a caring father. Two jobs, one that I must do and the other that I can enjoy. I am enjoying it now too, he is getting along fine and we do not fight.

Don't get me wrong, he struggles. Getting a job for instance. As an SP provider I can get him work. Due to his psychosis though he crumbles under pressure so getting him a job through a competitive interview is very difficult indeed. Then there are the problems around his disability. A frontline public service failed to renew his work placement there recently, implicitly because of his disabilities, they would not provide the necessary equipment or facilities for him to work there.

++++++++++++++++++++++

A note on stigma at work. A recent study shows that only 16% of people with Down's Syndrome will get a job[17], and this is no mental illness! Only the innocent, or employers of a good legal team, would *explicitly* deny someone a job because of

---

[17] Article claiming this on the Down's Syndrome website http://www.downs-syndrome.org.uk/DSA_detCampaign.aspx?cam=12

their disability with the raft of new legislation in place. In my case I nearly got a job with a US news agency but they had smart lawyers who made sure I couldn't take them to court.

In a list of interviewees the fittest for the job will win the job, and if the employer implicitly means that this is because someone's fitness is less so because of their disability, then they need to back this up with reasoning that is above the law before they refuse the job to the disabled.

In this way, far fewer disabled people get a sexy settlement from employment tribunals than should actually receive the money and headline media coverage of "Don't screw the disabled". Ian faced this with a father of attitude that he would take issue at Court, but knew the high risk of failure so did not. Disability discrimination runs rife in this country, law or no law.

++++++++++++++++++++++++++

Getting a job is important. Having a reason to get up in the morning is bread and butter necessary for someone in the world, but it really screws your head up if you don't have that. I saw it in Ian, both before he got that work placement and during, his mood changed for the better and overall he required less support and care. Why? For three afternoons a week he had to be at work. For three afternoons a week he had colleagues who knew him by name, and for those afternoons he had something to do. He's regressing again without it, though not anything like to the point he was at before we got him into his flat. There's something called the Disability Equality Duty which means employers must provide what's necessary for the employee to work, and that makes it somewhat harder to get employment in the first place as people see the accessibility issues for this employee and baulk.

I look to you Rich and realise you have a professional qualification and can be competitive in an interview, both with your CV and in the workplace. Ian has no such thing as an MA and frankly would not survive the lightest of interviews so I must find him a way of getting work without being interviewed. This is the bulk of my SP support given him now.
++++++++++++++

Horse shit. I am writing a book and running a media consultancy because I have been discriminated against in the workplace and know for a fact that I cannot be discriminated against as an employee of myself. I was cock sure that I could get a job threatening court action against discriminatory employers and this has been thoroughly disabused of me. I have no advice for the reader here, other than do your best and if you fail, start up your own business as many authors have at Chipmunka!

++++++++++++++++++

John rejoins…

Another form of support we provide is getting him out to the pub to play skittles. Again, getting Ian a life. His friends at that place are quite a bit older than him but he gets along well. Going out to the pub every week and having a work placement. An equation for you –

Same people + friendly faces = something to do

= happier, more stable,

= less care and support required.

For this level of SP I have to go before a tribunal every so often. The tribunal is required because he gets a high level of support. Supporting People is generally for people who require low level support. Ian might have difficulties in the night which fall under the support needs, so he can require 24/7 support. SP is generally for people who might need, say two or three hours a week as you got in your Second Step property. Under the rules he must be assessed periodically to ensure that my provision under the grant scheme is for his support needs and not for care.

I'll mention his care needs again... These are provided too, helping with the stuff his CP disables him from, physiotherapy for his CP... For this a separate payment system is in place called Direct Payments. Briefly this is money for specific needs he has that the state could provide but not of the consistency or same level of ability as the private sector. This is money given by the State for his care. As an SP provider I can ensure he administers those payments and does not lose his care. So he gets care from SP insofar as it enables him to get that money from his accounts into those of his care providers'. This also applies to his rent.

Cuts are mooted. What happened was a number of local authorities took SP with both hands and really used it. In this way the pot from THB became so large. However other authorities took little or no notice of the scheme, and thus there was not an equal distribution of funds across the UK. The Rt Hon Gordon Brown MP is an egalitarian, and this is a major factor in the mooted cuts, the idea being that the same pot is going to be redistributed across the UK equally. For this region, which took the piss in its approach to SP, it could mean a 30% cut. What should happen is that the SP budget should go up but the Treasury would weep as the already over doubled budget could go through an already high roof!

This is not due to the stigma of mental illness. That would be unequal, all those people receiving SP would suffer equally whilst the others not in receipt would benefit. Robbing the rich to give to the poor to cliché the catchphrase of the UK's most famous socialist!"
++++++++++++++++++

What would this mean to John and Ian? John would then be available to Ian for 16 hours a week, and extra time available to support his son would be either pro bono or reduced altogether. What Ian, and indeed the bulk of those in receipt of *SP* need is a lot of work initially to get them some momentum followed by a sloughing off of support.

Humans do not work to a bureaucratic timetable, despite the urging of the State to do so[18].

It might take two years or it might take five to get them rolling. In Ian's case, there'll always be a need of low level support for his cerebral palsy or any relapse in his psychosis. Funding that support is essential, or he might as well move either back in with his parents or with his sister for them to take his independence away altogether and firefight their way through to his parents' overworked, unhappy early death, and an unhappy, stressful, constrained rest of his own life.

When one engenders cerebral palsy, one thinks of a curled up man in a wheelchair surrounded by parents (until they die) and or a care team looking after him all day. Add a disorder such as psychosis and you get a grim picture of yelling and shouting, as well as dependency and care. Thanks to the will and fearlessness of John Wallace in the face of doubters and bureaucrats, Ian has a life. Able to stand and move around

---

[18] A chestnut so old the most starving of squirrels would not touch it

without aid in the first place, Ian was not cursed with his CP. But psychosis is an illness that can debilitate the individual to an equal degree to the stereotype engendered by Cerebral Palsy. Psychosis is a disabling illness and a killer in its own right, unless properly managed.

I now look to my aunt with Multiple Sclerosis. Wheelchair bound, and under the care of her Cinderella daughter. Direct Payments and the support of the NHS and Social Services provide a level of care that would not be found in a society such as the US but her daughter still has no life to speak of, I refer to Wendy as Cinderella for that very reason. She is a similar case to thousands of people in the UK young and old, who spend time and energy on a paltry income (£46 a week Carer's Allowance, from the Department of Work and Pensions) not out of direct volition but out of love for their family member.

John has escaped this confinement with his son. He found his way through barriers (that eventually closed behind him) to provide not only support for his son, but a means of breaking free from provision and care into a life of near independence and a fulfilled existence for John and Cathy *as well as* Ian. Most importantly for the bean counters in the Treasury this barrier should perhaps be dealt with for the simple reason that the Cinderellas of the world can make a positive contribution to society, instead of taking a poverty income which compares not at all with the Minimum Wage.

Thankfully there's politics here. One person in fifty in Bristol get support from *SP*, which taken to the UK is around a million people. They are of the poorest stratum of society, and amount to several constituencies of traditionally Labour loyal voters. The government therefore has trodden carefully and quietly – no headline grabbing here, just smooth movements that confound the eyesight of the Meerkat media.

SP is not currently a statutory funding provision of the same type as Housing Benefit is, no legal duty exists to provide it. The upshot is that the funding stream is voluntary and is not always provided by local authorities. Some ran with it and others ignored, generally the West of England took the Mickey with it as John said. Making *SP* a statutory fund would make provision compulsory, a boost for inequality and the so-called postcode lottery of services in our Welfare State. However, being centrally funded and thus administered would enable the government to cut it back and meddle. The classic case is the redistribution mooted above, where John would lose a third of his income. More likely than what the dreamers wish the bean counters to provide (the same services provided as now across the UK), this is just one of the possibilities *Supporting People* and the million odd clients could face.

The *Robson Rhodes LLP Report* looked at the scheme in some depth at a national level because the government wanted to know why it had so badly underestimated the budget required for *Supporting People*. Two headlines emerge, and this graph copied from the *Report* shows what the problem was[19].

Exhibit 4

The regional allocation per head of population shows a wide variation across authorities within the regions. At face value this analysis supports Ministers concern about the uneven distribution of the grant. However, at the median level the distribution looks more even for most regions.

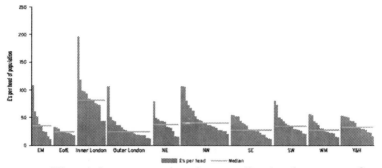

- There is a massive inequality in the use of funds nationwide and this is not because of the cost of regional centres, for instance "London weighted costs". A further breakdown of services provided, and not reprinted here, suggests similar variations in costs for mental health.

- This imbues a problem of efficiency – why is the unit cost of supporting someone in London less than a person of the same support needs in Newcastle?

In 2004 an article was published on SITRA website which said that the disinterested observer

---

[19] Robson Rhodes LLP Report, 2004

cannot look at a funding system such as this and say that it is fairly and evenly distributed:

"… what does government consider to be the 'right' distribution of SP monies? Certainly the current situation is hard to defend to people outside the sector. There are massive variations in SP Grant levels between regions, sub regions and even neighbouring local authorities which share very similar characteristics. For instance, two neighbouring inner London councils, with a long history of joint working received £40m and £17.5m in legacy funding respectively. "[20]

Even in London, one administering authority gets more than double what its neighbour got. This cannot be fair. However since the money is distributed according to what is applied for, a simple answer might be there may be less dribbling schizophrenics and incontinent grannies than the next borough?

This is a theme I shall return to later. I must move on, where more detail will help the reader understand the position I come to at the end of this chapter.

What of the property in which I lived? I had some good years, doing things that perhaps I needed to have done as a 20 year old student. Second Step is one of Bristol's largest supported housing providers, supporting about 1000 people in the

---

[20] Full article seen here
http://www.sitra.org.uk/index.php?id=712

city, or around one in five of those receiving support under SP.

It specialises in mental health. Several shared houses are in place for family sized groups of men and women receiving mental health care in the city. As discussed in *Andrew* the Director dreams of eventually supplanting the need for hospitalisation, providing support in daily living for the mental service users in its remit.

To me this meant having coffee with someone to shoot the breeze initially. Lesley Greig and later, Ruth Mayes became "paid friends" for a while, and are of those people one looks back to with fondness in the way I remember my A Level Biology teacher at school. To another housemate it meant getting to the shops, a lift to Sainsbury's and work with him on the budget so he didn't spend too much on beer and too little on potatoes! To us all it meant tidying the communal areas to a level dictated by Health and Safety, the "fire door" to the living room was not obstructed, but discord in the house was reduced by having a good hoover and a clean every week.

Aileen Edwards is introduced in the chapter *Andrew*, has been Director of Second Step since 1993. I spoke to her about the funding system under which Second Step operates.

Our funding up to 2001 was a hotchpotch of grants and statutory funding. Housing Benefit covered rent and some of our staffing costs. The

Housing Corporation gave us a grant. Social Services paid us from their Mental Health Fund, and a few other sources covered our requirements. Supporting People's remit was to consolidate all these funds into one stream and thereby cut fundraising time to a minimum, to pay us to do our work and not worry.

This came as a great relief to us, as it seemed that we were guaranteed our income for the long term, at a level that would provide for our clients comfortably. The government department running it at the time, the ODPM, promised us that we could expand our network and service provision too – this was a genuine golden opportunity and recognition of the work we do. It was coherent too, so supported housing providers had a clear remit and would be able to provide focussed services.

At the time we had around 400 clients in a range of support needs and service provision. Our immediate response was that we could expand our remit and the extent of our services. Prior to SP we worked in mental health and homeless resettlement provision. We now work in drug rehabilitation, have a floating support team, as well as our various supported accommodation in and around the Bristol area; we have expanded outside the Bristol authority to South Gloucestershire.

The system works, for every £1 spent on housing support through SP, 90 pence is saved in the area in which that support it given. In the mental health world, this means 90 pence saved by the NHS on a service user's non hospitalisation, 90 pence in drug rehab, 90 pence by the police…

The effects however came as a shock to the government. The original estimate fell well below the eventual costs and the State reacted by promising cuts immediately. This has not happened but things have not been so comfortable as a result. With threatened cuts of 30% and a definite grant freeze from the outset, how can an organisation plan strategically? We can work with the devil we know, that 75% of our income will not increase at the rate of inflation, we can expand our services according to service provision need, but we cannot guarantee for instance, that our staff would get hikes in their income according to inflation and the job market.

In March 2003 a report came out on the state of housing support in the UK, called the Robson Rhodes Report. This stated that though a number of Administering Authorities (the groups within councils that administer SP) worked well, efficiencies of output could be made in the system. This meant less bureaucracy and a slimmed down management system. To achieve this, we have had to increase our efficiency of output year on year.

++++++++++++++++++++++++

At this stage, we should remember that *Supporting People* is about people! There are two basic strands to *SP*, the people strand and the monitoring strand. The latter is a structure that must be in place to maintain standards of output. Looking into the history of asylums in the UK, in the 1800's asylums below a certain size did not have to undergo inspection and monitoring by the State. With hospitals such as Bedlam already known to have disgusting conditions, what would the small private asylums have been like? We just don't know[21].

Monitoring is essential in any service provision. There are two types, performance monitoring and the Quality Assurance Framework. The former has been shown to be inaccurate, with over 60% of the information submitted to the government claimed incorrect by Aileen. The latter assesses the quality of the services. Aileen refers to Second Step's approach to this as being "rigorous", quite rightly since when *SP* came into being loud murmurs of "paperwork" came from the staff on the front line!

Even John Wallace, with his single client service provision, must have a quality assurance and performance monitoring system in place. In an email he refers to this as being one of the structures that deters other single client operations from completing their approach to getting *SP* status:

Parents now face 4 or 5 problems:

---

[21]Listen to my documentary on asylums in the 1700's at http://www.b200fm.com/Lunacy.htm. A half hour show.

a. They would have to demonstrate that their service was strategically relevant and finance was available from the SP budget

b. They would have to demonstrate that the service was of high quality (comply with the Quality Assurance Framework and new contract conditions etc)

c. They would have to demonstrate that the service offered value for money

d. They would probably need strong support from Social Services to the effect that they represented the best option.

e. The accommodation issue needs to addressed - rented property with no security of tenure is not ideal for a long term service although a floating support service could possibly be offered.
++++++++++++++++++++++++++++

However, this doesn't approach the levels of bureaucratic insensibility that has been reported from other sectors of health and social provision; Second Step still provide a service and to my experience, do that job well. On the ground, QAF means that a support programme must be agreed with the client on a six to twelve month basis which might be a pain in the arse but really amounts to two hours of one week of the available 26 in that half year cycle.

The government would like to measure on a cost benefit or similar model, the success of supported housing. Was my 5 years in the Bristol house effective? Okay, so I won an MA but struggled hard to readjust to the real world after a prolonged spell in support. How do you quantify that? The MA knocks the success off the scale but even so getting a job (this book) 18 months after completing the course takes you down the scale. 6 months of outright schizophrenia too. I am somewhere around 5 on a scale of 1-10. My long suffering housemate "Matt", who moved in a month before me and out a month after, fared less well in that he has Grand Mal schizophrenia, is nocturnal and is unlikely to be fit to get a job for the rest of his life. Okay, with Grand Mal you change the scale some and state that when completely cuckoo he didn't wash or feed himself for 6 months. Therefore to smell deodorant and to see combed hair one afternoon (daylight) and weight gain, raises him up the scale – a 7 or 8. I am a 5 on my scale. What do these figures mean?

The government likes to know the effect of its money on the life of the person it funds to support. The QAF approach is leaning toward an "outcomes based approach". In Matt's situation this would mean that he goes to the shops independently and without support. In my case it would mean I am earning a living, but we're still talking two different scales; you cannot measure someone who had difficulty getting out of the house on the same scale as someone who found difficulty in getting a one year MA!

Performance monitoring is essential in monitoring the work of the service provider. It is extremely difficult to achieve; one could cite the National Institute of Health and Clinical Excellence and its cold measure of the cost benefit of keeping someone alive[22].

Aileen rejoins on the overall QAF framework.

Every six months there is a review of our output. We are graded on an A-D scale, where D is threatened grant withdrawal and A is very good. The monitoring is of the paperwork generated by the support provision, as well as the support plans of the clients. The support plans are a system of what the service user hopes to achieve in the next six months, and these are reviewed in terms of what has been achieved in that support plan, a significant step for instance is to go grocery shopping unsupported.

The accountability is based on the complexity of the paperwork; the thing that works best is a simple monitoring system and this is encouraged by the government. There are still reams of it involved and this brings about the duality of the "support agency" and the "government supported-support agency", where the "government

---

[22] How to measure the health effects of my antipsychotic Olanzipine? I am alive after 7 years but predominantly due to not committing suicide or having the stimulus to do so, the stimulus being irrelevant to the administration of the drug!

supported" part means relentless performance monitoring.

As we modify and simplify to accord value for money so we must embrace technology. Members of staff who are very good support workers may have neglected the Information Age in their pursuit of their careers, which were originally technology free. To that extent a number of them baulk at email circulars, let alone computerised QAF systems [even mobile phones for some!].

With the latest buzzword in the NHS being "payment by results", you can see that performance monitoring could soon directly equate with output. In a situation where the Foundation Hospital gets more money because it was of the best tranche in the first place and the lower grade hospital suffers and gets less cash, this is a policy future we have to be aware of and do well to eventually work within.

+++++++++++++++

I come in again with the emerging system that the government is suggesting at present. If there is such a variation in costs of support nationwide that doesn't correlate to the geography of the area, £17.5 million to one authority and £40 million to its next door neighbour for instance, why not allocate £3000 per head and give them that budget to pay for their support? (£3000 being the average on the graph detailed in *figure 1*) This would mean that the person receiving support would have a budget, per head and not per authority. From where I sit right now, this seems like a scheme that could work.

Variations emerge. Ian Wallace (see above) and I were in supported housing. He has 24/7 support needs and I had 3 hours a week of support needs. Thus, in this suggestion, give each person in receipt of funds a grading in the same way as disability benefits. I would get a lower level of support needs than Ian so he would have a higher support budget than me.

This is one of the suggestions being considered by the Department of Communities and Local Government at present, though it appears to a lower level of complexity.
For the moment there is confusion and some difficulty in strategic planning on the part of *SP* providers because while the government deliberates, it deliberates in silence, and you cannot write a business plan with silence as a policy document!

Second Step is a great housing provider and a wonderful place to work. This is the impression I have of the attitudes of staff there. Aileen closes her involvement in this chapter to give her line on this...

Second Step, with stout working procedures and management policy, has a good reputation in the Bristol area. We provide a service that people like from both a service user and policy maker's stance. As such we have been able to expand rapidly over the last few years, over doubling in size since SP came into being. We keep costs down without overworking our staff; I believe people feel it is a good organisation to work for. Budgetary freeze means that we constantly look for efficiency savings in our output, which has made us a cost effective service.

There is competition with the big guys. John Wallace refers to us as a big guy but there are national bodies that provide support across the UK, which make us look like a minnow. These aren't always playing the game, for instance some might claim that the elements not covered by SP are entirely met by charitable fundraising, the truth stretched I suspect, which may be seen as terrific efficiency and a level above that which Second Step could achieve.

As to the future? You relate how you had difficulty in re-engaging with society after receiving Second Step's support. Imagine that to be the case for 300 people in Second Step properties, some who are recent drug users, and others who avoid long stays in mental hospitals… It would be a disaster for the community should we see 30% of the funds we use redistributed to local authorities who did not take up the offer of Supporting People as much as Bristol.

For now, we hope we can meet the challenges ahead. We had a three year contract (that is coming to a close) to provide the services we do, we'd like to be on a longer contract but that hasn't offered because of government indecision. The best option I see is the status quo, with uncertainty being the shadow beneath the cloud. The worst option is not something we like to consider but we have to.

++++++++++++++++++++

With these allegations and uncertainties on the part of two South West *SP* providers, I approached the Department for Communities and Local Government for an interview. I appear to need to build my reputation before speaking to John Prescott, so was happy to receive a government statement as the response to four of five questions put to them.

1. Why have Administering Authorities been forced to freeze funding? In the three years to date, there has been no inflationary increase in funding.

In the lead up to Supporting People going live in 2003 the estimated costs of the programme increased by £400m.[23] The following Independent Review of the programme stated that the final costs of the programme (£1.8bn) were too much to pay for the inherited legacy services. Further work demonstrated that efficiencies could be found from the programme. All authorities between 2003 and April 2006 were required to review their SP funded services.

---

[23] Different parties, different figures. I side with the £1 billion as suggested by John Wallace; Aileen Edwards did not argue with this.

Through the review process many authorities have achieved efficiencies. This is demonstrated by the requests received from authorities to roll forward (within the SP programme) the efficiencies they have achieved into the following year. Day to day management of the programme is the responsibility of the local SP team - some authorities have chosen to pay inflation and others not- this is a local decision.

+++++++++++++++++++++++++

One might question why the Administering Authorities were so keen to continue the cuts. This sounds like manoeuvring to achieve the best deal they could get given limited options. John Wallace comments on this after this interview.

++++++++++++++++++++++++++++++++

2. There has been word that a redistribution of funds might take place in the year ahead. This would mean that organisations and authorities already in receipt of funding will lose out whilst authorities and organisations not presently in receipt would get funding from a pot that has not increased in size. Is this a rumour or a serious consideration for the new contracts?

As we stated when the funding allocations for 2007/08 were announced a decision has been taken to carry out further work on the analysis of responses to the consultation on the Supporting People distribution formula with a view to taking forward work on how we can distribute future funding based on need. We received a significant response to the consultation on the strategy and also the separate consultation on the formula which require further work, as outlined in the 'Next Steps' document

The formula is just one option that is being considered. No decision has been taken on what is the preferred approach.

++++++++++++++++++++++++

The Next Steps document is available on the SPK Web website[24]. To give detail, 600 recipients of *SP* and 400 organisations gave response to four consultation papers on the future of Supporting People. This is no stab in the dark on the part of the government. It raised the idea of looking at individual budgets for each person in receipt, passed from central government down. It led to, as will be discussed below, the budget proposal for 2007 – 2008.

We return to the final two questions answered by the government.

+++++++++++++++

3. Why has there been no increase in the overall pot if Supporting People is to be rolled out nationwide?

same answer as given in 1) above

---

[24] The Next Steps document is available on this website
http://www.spkweb.org.uk/NR/rdonlyres/AAFD8115-60ED-4060-9DE3-29D95E882F29/9864/SPstrategyWayForwardDocument.pdf

4. Why has there been dithering in decision making in regards Supporting People? Organisations I have dealt with have complained that they are incapable of making strategic plans because they cannot budget beyond the end of their next contract. This cannot help the people this is meant to provide stable and secure housing for, the socially excluded groups in the UK?

This is not the case. It has always been the intention of the SP programme to better target funding on the basis of need. The development of a Supporting People formula has been ongoing for a number of years and has now been used to limited degree to help inform grant allocations. At the time of announcing the 2007/08 grant allocations last summer it was announced that we would carry out further analysis on the responses to the technical paper on the formula and other responses to the Strategy about funding approaches. It is our intention to make a three year funding announcement once the SR07 settlement is agreed which will help authorities plan their provision of services in future years.

++++++++++++++++++++

I am clearly not the first person to ask this last question! In an article written for the SITRA website in 2004 for instance, Nigel Rogers raises the very same issue[25]. It again raised the issue of distribution of funds, which I quoted above[26].

What would the *SP* providers think of this response from the government? I approached John Wallace for his angle on it. I reproduce his email in full here:

1. The Treasury has insisted on a reduced SP pot and hence the Local Authority grants are in decline in most areas. In some areas, the costs have been transferred back to Social Services, particularly where 24/7 care is needed (back to the Care/Support debate). However areas such as North Somerset which did not go in for wholesale transfer of care to the THB/SP budget have still suffered.

2. With budgets in decline LA's cannot do much to increase service provision unless they tip Council Tax money into the SP pot. They are generally reluctant to do that (but are quite happy to pay extra money for SP admin costs which are subject to a separate grant) because it affects council tax.

At present the Treasury can get away with fixed budgets because SP funding is not a statutory right. With the advent of Individual Budgets for those who are disabled that position will become increasingly difficult to sustain but it might result in

---

[25] This article is shown on the SITRA website at http://www.sitra.org.uk/index.php?id=712

[26] Quoted from SITRA website in previous pages. See full article referenced in footnote 25

more cuts for those who are not disabled but need help.

Council Tax. The tax that gives local councillors the right to speak on politics, yet only covers a quarter of Local Authority budgets. LA's have the right to increase their *SP* budgets providing they can source that funding from elsewhere. In most cases this means from the much maligned community charge. Bristol City Council once put a Council Tax raise to referendum in the city to ask whether they should raise the Education budget and Bristolians pay for it. Bristol voted - No! In this way the government says that the non statutory scheme is administered by Local Authorities, and in theory it is an open pot to which anyone may add funds. In practice, this is emphatically not the case; there are far more electorally appealing things to raise Council Tax for (such as recycling and other rubbish)!

At the time of writing, the budget for the next two years is out for *SP*. Bristol loses money, around £1 million on last year's budget, about 300 people losing support overall (though unlikely to happen. More like all 5000 will get 5% less support). If one looks at the nationwide budget allocations[27], you will see that Bristol is a big player in *SP*. One of the measures suggested in this chapter as making

---

[27] Budget allocations are detailed in this letter from the DCLG, to be found in Annex A of this site http://www.spkweb.org.uk/NR/rdonlyres/36DFA59C-2B08-4C66-AC1D-70F8FE8D0AA1/7189/051202FundingAnnouncement1.doc

sense for individuals is the *Individual Budget* system. In theory this would provide the person with choice in the support and care he or she receives, giving them the money to pay for that support and letting them employ the providers themselves. Simply put, the pilot hopes to:

enable people needing social care and associated services to design that support and to give them the power to decide the nature of the services they need. Key features are:

- A transparent allocation of resources, giving individuals a clear cash or notional sum for them to use on their care or support package

- A streamlined assessment process across agencies, meaning less time spent giving information

- Bringing together a variety of streams of support and/or funding, from more than one agency.

Giving individuals the ability to use the budget in a way that best suits their own particular requirements[28]

So, rather than being told by my Social Worker that there was a house for me to move into and that I should take all the services provided there, I may have seen that I wanted a shared house to

---

[28] Link to this document to be found for the best explanation on the Web for Individual Budgets, http://individualbudgets.csip.org.uk/index.jsp

live in, and been given the budget for that with Housing Benefit paying. Then, 3 hours support a week, a budget for that...

This is very much the way the government leans at present, putting money with the individual and letting them get the best care and support they need. A similar system lies in place for care, the Direct Payment scheme, referred to in my chats with John Wallace earlier on in this chapter. Why then, should this not be used?

A consultation response document from another area of the Supporting People scheme, this time a women's refuge network in Wolverhampton, suggests that this might not always be the answer[29].

Individual Budgets
We believe that individual budgets are not appropriate or applicable for our client group. Our service users are at a crisis point in their lives and some may not have the ability to handle managing individual budgets as well as their circumstances. There is also a concern that individual budgets could lead to exclusion for some services users who may be unable to find a provider who is prepared to work with them. We predict that individual budgets for our client group will be extremely difficult to manage.

---

[29] Quoted from webpage
http://www.havenrefuge.org.uk/Consultations/SP%20Strateg
y%20Response%20Haven.doc

GIVING VOICE TO THE INNER SCREAM

In crisis, you might not be able to work with this scheme. I would hazard my friend with Grand Mal schizophrenia would struggle too. In fact, the way this is being put, nor would a large chunk of those receiving the money – severe mental illness, drug problems (where a £10er in the wallet is a fire in the belly down the pub), even a fading OAP who struggles already with her pension being paid electronically. You'd need Direct Payments for the "care" to run your budget and pay people on time, and thus manage your budget for "support" in Individual Budgets. The clear headed writer gets confused at this, let alone a freaked out schizophrenic with a pen in one hand and chequebook the other! A pilot is being run over 13 authorities, the results to be heard in 2008, so for the moment we shall hear in good time what the decision of the government, and the providers think.

As is *Supporting People* works. Some may argue that it needs bedding in before it works as effectively as it might. Others may argue that it needs radical cuts. My own impression is that it came as a shock to the government that so many people would require so much support, so it is trying to shave it back. A message to all Meerkat journalists here, keep your eyes on it or it might just be Sweeney Todd Barbers Ltd, (*by Royal Appointment to HM The Treasury*) shaving it still further…

A mad world...

First things first – go read him. Go and read *Fear and Loathing in Las Vegas, Hell's Angels,* and preferably two or three of the "best of" books, the *Gonzo Papers.* This man was a first class writer who had adventures that I often wished for in my own wayward path, and lived life on the edge. Who doesn't wish for experiences on the edge, crossing the boundaries set by "normal society" and enjoyed the more for it?

I for one, think anyone who has got a First Class at university, never had more than a couple of pints down the pub, never smoked a joint and walked away debt free at the end of your twenties, is boring.

I relate my own life throughout this book. Do I regret what led to getting paranoid schizophrenia? I regret getting the illness, but not before or after. If you don't climb the odd fence in life then you have wasted it. Unless you're climbing the fence that says "only the most boring in here", go ahead and climb it.

The boring person will see another angle; they did not have miserable formative years. I relate how I hated school at the time. But I enjoyed a lot of it. Running half marathons at a rate of 5 minute miles and lower, sailing, even being interrogated by the Deputy Headmaster...

GIVING VOICE TO THE INNER SCREAM

Pope Benedict was a Hitler Youth as a youngster. If he had gone the opposite way as an adult (and forgotten his right wing views) I might even respect him. As is, to rise from something most regard as an evil little Boy Scout to being considered the holiest man in the world by a billion people, ain't a bad path to follow. Good on you Popey (now go tell people that condoms prevent AIDS you Nazi bastard).

In Hunter S Thompson's memoirs[30], an aged ex hippy asked the man, "how did you survive?" reflecting his drug use throughout his life, and the experiences had as a result. Most people, and particularly those people who have not come away unscathed, would ask that of Thompson.

He was one of the most famous hedonists the world has seen. He related things that many people have done in vivid detail and has done some of the most extreme things that a man can do to his nervous system. In a world where we earn money *to* get blasted in our twenties, this man earned a living *from* getting blasted throughout his life!

The boring person will read this another way. Thompson (aka, HST) was a loser who found nothing better to do than write weird ramblings while out of his head on DMT, LSD, Mescaline, Mandrax... Okay you boring bugger (hence known as BB), go do it. I did and cracked up, you do the

---

[30] HST (2003) *Kingdom of Fear,* Penguin

same and unless you're lucky, you will be a loony too. Hunter S Thompson was in the right place at the right time and not only made a living doing what he found pleasurable, but made a mint doing it.

However I want to relate this argument in the following pages. For someone so obviously cheering the leadership of this man into the abyss, I am going to rebel again. I am now boring.

I wanted to take the angle of the BB because something needs to be shown – that the two labels of "madness" are interchangeable. Society stigmatises the unusual, the feared. The streaker who runs across the lawns at Wimbledon, showing his knackers to the world before being arrested, is laughed with and often makes a dull and depressing match with Henman snatching defeat from the jaws of victory worth watching. The same man who drops his clothes at a church fete is considered a sick weirdo, even if the old women there were titillated by the first sight of prick in the twenty years since menopause.

Hunter S Thompson committed suicide in 2003. This would suggest that contrary to the position that he had survived years of drug abuse, he did not. What made him top himself? In his suicide note[31] he alluded he had done all he wanted to do in life and that the time was right to end it. Ralph

---

[31] Suicide note covered in the Wikipdedia entry on HST. Read it at this address:
http://en.wikipedia.org/wiki/Hunter_S._Thompson

GIVING VOICE TO THE INNER SCREAM

Steadman relates in *The Joke's Over,* how Thompson had made a decision early on that he would not die by natural causes, and providing that nothing else got him first, he would choose to end it himself. In most walks of life, suicide is committed because the person has apparently insurmountable problems and in a state of depression decides to end it all. According to this idea, did Thompson die because of underlying mental illness?

I approached Dr Stanley Zammit, introduced in the chapter *Andrew*, with a "standardised patient" for him to come up with a diagnosis of the illnesses that Mr Thompson might have had.

Here's the initial email and the standardised patient[32]...

Stan

Attached is a 6 page case study on the writer I am studying. Three pages are a summary of his life and behaviour, with two excerpts of his writing, another 3 pages.

At the bottom of page 3 is the section **Possible Causes**. These are the questions I ask. On receipt of the conclusions drawn I will send another page

---

[32] References in Standardised Patient added after submission to the doctor – they're in for journalistic propriety and were not included for anonymity of the subject to be maintained in this experiment.

or so with an update to see if this matches the conclusions to your mind.

Cheers

R

Diagnosis request.

The subject, hence known as Robert, is being referred by a fellow writer because he is worried about the man's behaviour, lifestyle and habits. Robert is a 67 year old white male with a history of drug abuse who has been referred for assessment for multiple concerns about his behaviour, beliefs and actions. These include substance abuse, extreme beliefs, risk taking, and aggressive, threatening behaviour.

History of the present illness

Robert was expelled from school without matriculating. Jailed in the 1950's for armed robbery, after some years drifting between jobs, he became a journalist. This started a stunning career and he is now a millionaire with a ranch in the Rocky Mountains in the US.

Despite his success, he has had frequent brushes with the law ranging from driving while under the influence to accusations of sexual assault and firearms offences. He has abused drugs, he is known to drink brandy from first thing in the morning and takes a large amount of illegal narcotics.

He has been married twice and has a son by the first marriage. Family life is good, though friendships and work relationships have been suffering.

Known medical information

He drinks brandy constantly. He does this from the time he gets up in the morning. He is well known to drink whilst driving. A close friend describes his method for drinking beer, brandy, and smoking marijuana simultaneously whilst at the wheel[33].

He regularly snorts cocaine. It is known he uses this and other stimulants to start the day and uses marijuana and alcohol to help him sleep. Reports from family and friends suggest that his cocaine use is habitual[34].

In the 1960's and 70's he wrote accounts of taking large doses of hallucinogenic substances ranging from LSD to mescaline to DMT. See Extract of stream of consciousness account of a drugs trip.

Physical illnesses. He has had a range of medical problems over the years. Currently he has severe

---

[33] Ralph Steadman, (2006) *The Joke's Over* – memories of Hunter S Thompson Heinnemann

[34] Read anything on the man and you will read about drug use being recounted.

arthritis in his hands, and whole body shakes uncontrollably for reasons unknown.

Psychology

Robert has a persistent belief that the US Federal authorities will storm his house. Has had slam shut gates installed on driveway to home for protection and has an arsenal of firearms.

Temper volatile at best, prone to violent rages. People feel unsafe around him at times.

Has extreme political views. Hates neo-conservatism to an unusual degree. See Letter to editor of the UK Independent newspaper.

Destruction of own and others' property – use of TNT and plastic explosives at home to destroy property. Leaves hotel rooms in unusable state after vacating them.

Use of firearms. Prone to pointing a high powered handgun in peoples' faces in fit of temper. Fascination with weaponry bordering on obsessional. Recites the US Constitution to reinforce.

Sometimes incapable of making engagements, personal or otherwise, at times. Missed a Mohammed Ali fight in Zaire and a UK royal engagement despite being flown to both and being paid well.

GIVING VOICE TO THE INNER SCREAM

Sleep patterns non existent and unpredictable. May sleep all night and work all day or the reverse.

Relationships

Work.

Robert is an extremely talented writer in high demand by a range of publications worldwide. Has several factual and fiction books published. He is egocentric and proud of his achievements.

However his unpredictability and behaviour makes working with him extremely difficult at times. Sometimes he makes a print deadline with minutes to spare; at others this is not achieved.

His paymasters accept this as par for the course but dislike working with him – his name sells papers and magazines so have to put up with it for circulation.

Social relationships

Again, people are drawn to the legend of the man but repelled by the behaviour and unpredictability.

People are drawn to the unpredictability because it is fun but often this has had near fatal consequences – a close friend recounts drink driving and narcotic abuse situations that were frightening at the time but were "good to talk about in the pub after".

Prone to telling people to leave and never return from his life and then blame them for not contacting him.

<u>Personal relationships</u>

Robert has been married twice. Both were comfortable marriages, no remarked upon violence against the spouses. However he is a sexual predator and has had a string of affairs during this time. He was accused of rape but this was put down by the Courts to a malicious accusation.

<u>Family</u>

Robert had one son by his first marriage. The son put up with his father's behaviour but related that he did not look up to Robert as a role model.

Good relationship with mother, who has been treated for alcoholism. Relationship with rest of the family unknown.

Contact with mental health services

Occasional confrontations with services throughout life but never compulsorily treated.

Possible causes?

GIVING VOICE TO THE INNER SCREAM

With the available information, please could you offer possible diagnoses or conditions that could explain these behaviours before the chronic substance abuse?

Also, with your possible diagnoses what impact chronic substance and other medication abuse would have upon the possible diagnoses?

Appendix 1 – unknown chemical hallucinogen account[35].

Getting toward dawn now, very foggy in the head... and no Dexedrine left. For the first time in at least 5 years I am out of my little energy bombs. Nothing in the bottle but five Ritalin tablets and a big spansule of mescaline and "speed". I don't know the ratio of the mixture, or what kind of speed is in there with the mescaline. I have no idea what it will do to my head, my heart, or my body. But the Ritalin is useless at this point – not strong enough – so I'll have to risk the other. Oscar is coming by at ten, to take me out to the airport for the flight to Denver and Aspen...

Jesus, 6:45 now and the pill has taken hold for real. The metal on the typewriter has turned from dull green to a sort of high gloss blue, the keys sparkle, glitter with highlights... I sort of levitated in the chair, hovering in front of the typewriter, not sitting. Fantastic brightness on everything, polished and waxed with special lighting... and the

---

[35] HST (1990) Songs of the Doomed pp121-122 Picador

physical end of the thing is like the first half – hour on acid, a sort of buzzing all over, a sense of being gripped by something, vibrating internally but no outward sign of movement. I'm amazed that I can keep typing. I feel like both me and the typewriter have become weightless; it floats in front of me like a bright toy… Weird, I can still spell… but I had to think about this last one… "Weird". Christ, I wonder how much worse this is going to get. Its seven now, and I have to check out in an hour or so. If this is the beginning of an acid-style trip I might just as well give up on the idea of flying anywhere. Taking off in an airplane right now would be an unbearable experience, it would blow the top right off my head. The physical sensations of lifting off the ground would be unbearable in this condition; I feel like I could step off the balcony right now and float gently down to the sidewalk. Yes, and getting worse, a muscle in my thigh is seized by spasms, quivering like some disembodied… I can watch it, feel it, but not be connected. There is not much connection between my head and body… but I can still type and very fast too, much faster than normal. Yes, the goddamn drug is definitely taking hold, very much like acid, a sense of very pleasant physical paralysis (wow, that spelling), while the brain copes with something never coped with before. The brain is doing all the work right now, adjusting to this new stimulus like an old soldier ambushed and panicked for a moment, getting a grip but not in command, hanging on, waiting for a break but expecting something far worse… and yes, it's coming on. I couldn't possibly get out of this chair right now, I couldn't walk, all I can do is type… it feels like the blood is racing through me, all around me, at fantastic speeds. I don't feel any pumping, just an increased flow… Speed. Interior speed… and a buzzing without noise, high speed vibrations and more brightness. The little red indicator that moves along with the ball on this typewriter now appears to be made of arterial blood. It throbs and jumps along like a living thing.

Appendix 2 – Letter to the Editor of the Independent[36]

Dear Simon

Millions of people around the world are watching the headlines and most of them are getting the Fear. Good news is out of the question in this brutal year of our Lord 2002. This is the time of the Final Shit Rain, as Nostradamus predicted in 1444AD, and anybody who thinks he was kidding should strut out purposefully, like some all American girl with a head full of Mandrax and try to get a job in this country… Yes sir, little sweetie, just walk right up here and get what's coming to you. Ho ho ho.

There are no jobs in America, Simon; the job market collapsed in 2001 AD, along with the stock market and all ENRON pension funds. All markets collapsed about 3 days after George W Bush moved into the White House… Yeah, it was that

---

[36] HST (2003) Kingdom of Fear pp332 – 334 Penguin

fast. BOOM, presto, welcome to bombs and poverty. You are about to start paying for the sins of your fathers and forefathers, even if they were innocent.

We are in bad trouble over here, Simon. The deal is going down all over the once-proud USA. We are down to our last cannonballs(s). Stand back! Those Pentagon swine are frantic to kick some ass, and many job opportunities are opening up in the Armaments, Surveillance, and New Age Security industries.

Hell, did I forget to mention those jobs? How silly of me. There is always a bull market for vengeance and violence in America, and on some days I have been part of it. You bet. In my wild and dangerous youth I wanted to be a dashing jet pilot, a smiling beast who zooms across the sky doing victory rolls and monster sonic booms just over the beach in Laguna. Hot damn, Simon, I could walk on water in those days. I had a license to kill.

I have been a news addict all my life, and I feel pretty comfortable with my addiction. It has been good to me, although not necessarily for me, or my overall comfort level. Being a news junkie has taken me down some very queer roads, and into the valley of death a few times – not always for strictly professional reasons alas - but those things do come with the territory, and you want to understand this: It is the key to survival in my business, as it is in many others.

GIVING VOICE TO THE INNER SCREAM

And you definitely want to have a shockproof sense of humour, which is hard to learn in school and even harder to teach. (It is also an irritating phrase to keep putting on paper over and over – so from now on we will use the ancient and honourable word "WA" instead of "sense of humour". It will smooth out our word-rhythms and we can move along more briskly.)

Okay. We were talking about the news – information or intelligence gained from afar, etc, etc.

The news is bad today, in America and for America. There is nothing good or hopeful about it – except for Nazis, warmongers, and rich greedheads – and it is getting worse and worse in logarithmic progressions since the fateful bombing of the World Trade Towers in New York. That will always be a festering low water mark in this nation's violent history, but it was not the official birthday of the end of the American Century.

No. That occurred on the night of the presidential election in the year 2000, when the nexus of power in this country shifted from Washington DC to "the ranch" in Crawford, TX. The most disastrous day in American history was November 7, 2000. That was when the takeover happened when the generals and cops and right – wing Jesus freaks seized control of the White House, the US Treasury, and our Law Enforcement machinery.

So long to all that, eh? "Nothing will be the same again", the whorish new President said at the time. "As of now we are in the grip of a National Security Emergency that will last for the rest of our lives".

Fuck you. I quit. Mahalo.

I would never claim to speak for my whole nation, Simon; I am not the Voice of America – but neither am I a vicious machine-gun Nazi warmonger with blood on my hands and hate in my heart for every human being in he world who is not entirely white – and, if you wonder why I mention this thuggish characterization, understand that I am only responding to it in this way because my old friend… is saying these horrible things…

Ever since (I think) I talked to you on yr. birthday I have been feverishly writing down my various fears and worries and profoundly angst – ridden visions about our immediate future.

So good luck, Simon. Pls advise me at once re space & rates. How about $20 000, eh? I can ramble for many hours about my experience as an American these days at the end of our Century. Or maybe just 1000 words, or 2000. Think about it, and RSVP soonest.

Thanks.
++++++++++++++++
Dr Zammit responded thus:

GIVING VOICE TO THE INNER SCREAM

Rich

You don't know what his underlying problem was - was he very depressed? Was he psychotic? Was he drunk or drug intoxicated? Was he sadistic/psychopathic? any or all of those could have been operating to any degree.

I think most people would say he could have had any or all of the above, and drug/alcohol use would make ANY mental health problem worse

Stan.
+++++++++++++

Hunter S Thompson – depressed, psychotic, sadistic and psychopathic. Many fans of his get that idea when reading of his impulsive and crazy life events! Readers of HST's works will know that the excerpts above are some of his tamer recollections.

With this list, one can look up the symptoms of the illnesses and come up with a suggested diagnosis of Thompson. There are two lines of diagnosis used by psychiatrists around the globe, the *International Classification of Diseases and Related Health Problems, 10th Edition, (ICD-10)* which is published by the World Health Organisation, and the *Diagnostic and Statistical Manual of Mental Disorders, Fourth Edition (DSM –IV)* which is more often used in the United States. Debate as to which is the better manual for psychiatric use worldwide is often enacted in the more expert professional and psychiatric patients' world, and I will not enjoin it here. My criterion for which one to use was firstly ease of use – the ICD-10 is online and has its own website. Add in cost of use – the DSM is a book and has to be paid for whereas the ICD-10 is free to anyone who wants to refer to it. Simple enough choice!

Using the *ICD-10*[37] I show the various disorders described by Dr Zammit.

Diagnosis - Depression

F32 Depressive episode

In typical mild, moderate, or severe depressive episodes, the patient suffers from lowering of mood, reduction of energy, and decrease in activity. Capacity for enjoyment, interest, and concentration is reduced, and marked tiredness after even minimum effort is common. Sleep is usually disturbed and appetite diminished. Self-esteem and self-confidence are almost always reduced and, even in the mild form, some ideas of guilt or worthlessness are often present. The lowered mood varies little from day to day, is unresponsive to circumstances In typical mild, moderate, or severe depressive episodes, the patient suffers from lowering of mood, reduction of energy, and decrease in activity. Capacity for enjoyment, interest, and concentration is reduced,

---

[37] http://www.who.int/classifications/apps/icd/icd10online/

and marked tiredness after even minimum effort is common. Sleep is usually disturbed and appetite diminished. Self-esteem and self-confidence are almost always reduced and, even in the mild form, some ideas of guilt or worthlessness are often present. The lowered mood varies little from day to day, is unresponsive to circumstances and may be accompanied by so-called "somatic" symptoms, such as loss of interest and pleasurable feelings, waking in the morning several hours before the usual time, depression worst in the morning, marked psychomotor retardation, agitation, loss of appetite, weight loss, and loss of libido. Depending upon the number and severity of the symptoms, a depressive episode may be specified as mild, moderate or severe.

Conclusion

Thompson was not known for his lack of motivation – he did enough in life that being too down to get out of bed could not be attributed to him. Did he think himself worthless? He was an egotist, sure that people (like myself here) were using him to earn money off his back. Finally, he was known to have affairs as well as his relationships with his two wives, so libido was not an issue. We can conclude that he was not depressed.

Diagnosis - Mania

Was he a maniac? A description not mentioned by Dr Zammit but readily proffered to the man, though not necessarily with understanding. A maniac is defined in the Cambridge Dictionaries Online [38]

Maniac
noun *[C]*
a person who behaves in an uncontrolled way, not caring about risks or danger: Some maniac was running down the street waving a massive metal bar. INFORMAL I won't get in the car with Richard - he drives like a maniac!

This definition is in ready use as a description of a person. I am considered a maniac when I charge down the beach with a 7 square metre kite up in strong winds on my kite buggy, but laughingly so and the same person will buy me a Coke down the pub afterwards. Thompson was considered a maniac because he behaved in an uncontrolled way with almost everything he did; his drug use and behaviour with that drug use rising foremost in the eyes of the beholder of his actions.

What of the psychiatrist's viewpoint? Mania is something that has people locked up in mental hospitals. Mania is a dangerous illness,

---

[38]

http://dictionary.cambridge.org/define.asp?key=48587&dict=CALD

associated with colossal highs of happiness and suicidal lows. The ICD-10[39] describes it as

F30.1 Mania without psychotic symptoms

Mood is elevated out of keeping with the patient's circumstances and may vary from carefree joviality to almost uncontrollable excitement. Elation is accompanied by increased energy, resulting in over activity, pressure of speech, and a decreased need for sleep. Attention cannot be sustained, and there is often marked distractibility. Self-esteem is often inflated with grandiose ideas and overconfidence. Loss of normal social inhibitions may result in behaviour that is reckless, foolhardy, or inappropriate to the circumstances, and out of character.

F30.2 Mania with psychotic symptoms

In addition to the clinical picture described in F30.1, delusions (usually grandiose) or hallucinations (usually of voices speaking directly to the patient) are present, or the excitement, excessive motor activity, and flight of ideas are so extreme that the subject is incomprehensible or inaccessible to ordinary communication.

Conclusion

---

[39] See footnote 37 for the website

Here is where we leave Thompson and for the first time, go to a British city centre on a Friday night. People are found with mood "*out of keeping with the patient's circumstances*" and "*uncontrollable excitement*". Taking the BB's angle, why would people find so much excitement in a sweat smelling, steamy room with people behaving without control? What makes them so excited about going with their girlfriend to consume drugs that might wind up with the girlfriend sleeping with another man (or more than one)? Is this normal? The mania is considered normal because the mania is induced by a legal drug, alcohol.

Diagnosis - psychopathic

Psychopathic is a description given by Dr Zammit. Put in the website, ICD-10[40] spits out a range of disorders…

F07.0 <u>*Organic personality disorder*</u>

F21 <u>*Schizotypal disorder*</u>

F60.2 <u>*Dissocial personality disorder*</u>

Dissocial personality disorder comes up on the above link as

F60.2 *Dissocial personality disorder*

---

[40] ICD-10 website as in footnote 37

GIVING VOICE TO THE INNER SCREAM

Personality disorder characterized by disregard for social obligations, and callous unconcern for the feelings of others. There is gross disparity between behaviour and the prevailing social norms. Behaviour is not readily modifiable by adverse experience, including punishment. There is a low tolerance to frustration and a low threshold for discharge of aggression, including violence; there is a tendency to blame others, or to offer plausible rationalizations for the behaviour bringing the patient into conflict with society.

Personality (disorder):
· *amoral*
· *antisocial*
· *asocial*
· *psychopathic*
· *sociopathic*

Conclusion

Disregard for social obligations, the *Guardian* incident in the standardised patient above, tick. *Callous unconcern for the feelings of others*, his suicide with son as invited audience, tick. *Behaviour not readily modifiable by adverse experience* – most of his life, tick. In fact Thompson showed most of these symptoms in life. We will come back to this later with reference to Britain's city centres on a Friday night. For now, we'll plough on through the possible diagnoses that come from Dr Zammit.

Diagnosis - psychotic

Psychosis was another element suggested by Dr Zammit. Thompson famously related a Las Vegas policemen's convention entirely populated by lizards![41] This was drug induced, in the same way as Dr Zammit described that psychosis can be induced in a laboratory environment with the use of cannabis in the chapter, *Andrew*. Which drugs turned the policemen into lizards in this situation is not clear, but there was something involved...

Psychosis is one of the most stigmatised illnesses. I was not refused entry to the news organisation because of schizophrenia; I only related that I suffer from psychosis. I start by relating the Cambridge dictionary's version of psychosis[42]:

psychosis
noun [C or U] plural psychoses. Any of a number of the more severe mental diseases that make you believe things that are not real

A child believing in Father Christmas is psychotic to this definition!

The lizards described above were not real. Nor was the fact that the authorities were going to storm Thompson's house out of pure malice. (They'd consider storming for the drugs, explosives...)

---

[41] In *Fear and loathing in Las Vegas*
[42] http://dictionary.cambridge.org/

Let's look at the ICD-10[43] for definition of this set of symptoms.

F23 Acute and transient psychotic disorders

A heterogeneous group of disorders characterized by the acute onset of psychotic symptoms such as delusions, hallucinations, and perceptual disturbances, and by the severe disruption of ordinary behaviour. Acute onset is defined as a crescendo development of a clearly abnormal clinical picture in about two weeks or less. For these disorders there is no evidence of organic causation. Perplexity and puzzlement are often present but disorientation for time, place and person is not persistent or severe enough to justify a diagnosis of organically caused delirium (F05.-). Complete recovery usually occurs within a few months, often within a few weeks or even days. If the disorder persists, a change in classification will be necessary. The disorder may or may not be associated with acute stress, defined as usually stressful events preceding the onset by one to two weeks.

Conclusion

Hallucinations, tick. *Delusions*, tick. *Severe disruption of ordinary behaviour*. This last one lifts the lid on the difficulty of diagnosing Thompson because he was almost permanently cut on drugs of some form or other. How does one describe the

---

[43] Ibid footnote 37

departure from normal behaviour without knowing what normal behaviour in the case of the subject was?

This question was raised by Dr Zammit. Throughout our discussions he insisted he could not give anything hard and fast because HST was only known to me, a reader of his works and certainly no acquaintance of Thompson's, through his and others relating his experiences. Blasted on drugs, you can exhibit a range of psychiatric symptoms. I go on to suggest psychiatric diagnoses of the crowd in a British city centre on a Saturday night, but they are only exhibiting those symptoms – they are not diagnosable per se (except in some cases their substance misuse problems).

In his case, abnormal behaviour was known to be one of his more endearing nuances, people went to him for a crazy time. In concluding this chapter we shall draw conclusions, for the moment we shall move on to other potential diagnoses.

Diagnosis - schizophrenia

Many people with psychosis are given the label of schizophrenia, probably the most stigmatised illness of them all. Whereas I'd be slapped on the back and told "you maniac" after relating my 50mph journey down the beach under kite and on buggy, the same man would run away if I had said there were sharks chasing me down the beach, and that's why I was going so fast. This is symptomatic of some forms of schizophrenia, hallucinations. Dr Zammit did not describe the illness in reference to Thompson, but it is worth looking at here.[44]

F20 Schizophrenia

The schizophrenic disorders are characterized in general by fundamental and characteristic distortions of thinking and perception, and affects that are inappropriate or blunted. Clear consciousness and intellectual capacity are usually maintained although certain cognitive deficits may evolve in the course of time. The most important psychopathological phenomena include thought echo; thought insertion or withdrawal; thought broadcasting; delusional perception and delusions of control; influence or passivity; hallucinatory voices commenting or discussing the patient in the third person; thought disorders and negative symptoms.
The course of schizophrenic disorders can be either continuous, or episodic with progressive or stable deficit, or there can be one or more episodes with complete or incomplete remission. The diagnosis of schizophrenia should not be made in the presence of extensive depressive or manic symptoms unless it is clear that schizophrenic symptoms antedate the affective disturbance. Nor should schizophrenia be diagnosed in the presence of overt brain disease or during states of drug intoxication or withdrawal.

---

[44] Ibid footnote 33

Similar disorders developing in the presence of epilepsy or other brain disease should be classified under F06.2, and those induced by psychoactive substances under F10-F19 with common fourth character .5.

Excludes: schizophrenia:
· acute (undifferentiated) (*F23.2*)
· cyclic (*F25.2*)
schizophrenic reaction (*F23.2*)
schizotypal disorder (*F21*)

F20.0 Paranoid schizophrenia

Paranoid schizophrenia is dominated by relatively stable, often paranoid delusions, usually accompanied by hallucinations, particularly of the auditory variety, and perceptual disturbances. Disturbances of affect, volition and speech, and catatonic symptoms, are either absent or relatively inconspicuous.

Conclusion

Thompson could not be diagnosed with this illness for the simple reason he was intoxicated for most of the period he was known to have these behaviours…

Nor should schizophrenia be diagnosed in the presence of overt brain disease or during states of drug intoxication or withdrawal.

GIVING VOICE TO THE INNER SCREAM

As such one cannot describe Thompson, for all his whacko behaviours, as schizophrenic.

++
+++++++++++++++++++++++++++++++++

I was invited to Dr Zammit's office at Bristol University to discuss HST. There, he reinforced this last statement, that when you're out of your tree on drugs, you may simulate a range of psychiatric behaviours.

Take the 20 year old hedonist in a city centre. At work, she is a model citizen. At the office ten minutes early, works a full day and is held in high esteem by her workmates and boss for her output. Always well dressed to work, no unsightly creases from clothes left on the floor, no sign of the animal that she becomes when she goes out at 7 on Friday night with the intention of waking in a strange man's bed with hazy memory of how she got there. Of how she enjoyed the process of drinking so much booze her liver hangs by a thread, of her whooping loudly as her friend vomits on the street between pubs, and then loses yet more inhibition as she threatens another woman with a glass for trying her luck with her male target for the evening; "get your fucking hands off him, he's mine…"

As I discussed with Dr Zammit in the chapter, *Andrew*, psychoactive drugs are used to induce psychosis and other symptoms for laboratory analysis of these illnesses. It is known that a certain dose of cannabis will induce paranoia. What is borne out by the discussion of HST's life and outlook was that he was in such a haze of narcotics that the behaviours he exhibited (psychopathy, asocial personality, psychosis, depression…), were symptoms of the drug use.

The party continued for two days and nights but the only other crisis came when the worldly inspiration for the protagonist of several recent novels stood naked on the private side of the creek and screamed a long brutal diatribe against the cops only twenty yards away. He was swaying and yelling in a bright glare of a light from a porch, holding a beer in one hand and shaking his fist at the objects of his scorn: 'You sneaky motherfuckers! What the fuck's wrong with you? Come on over here and see what you get … God damned shit – filled souls anyway!' Then he would laugh and wave his beer around. 'Don't fuck with me you sons of shitlovers. Come on over. You'll get every fucking thing you deserve![45]

This example isn't too far from the average British city centre on a Friday night. The excerpt was of someone considered more respectable in most circles than your call centre weenie, he was a successful novelist. This party was held by a group of Beatniks and there was definitely drugs about, which imbues his inhibition was long gone. Particularly so since the people he was yelling at

---

[45] HST (1967) Hell's Angels, pp277 Penguin

was a group of California State Police intent on raiding the party!

After a few days, Dr Zammit returned the suggested diagnosis. This is to be found in the Appendix.

Conclusions to my understanding of Dr Zammit's suggestions.

Asocial personality disorder comes up twice in the responses from Dr Zammit. This was mentioned earlier on in this chapter. Again we shall quote the ICD-10[46]

F60.2 Dissocial personality disorder

Personality disorder characterized by disregard for social obligations, and callous unconcern for the feelings of others. There is gross disparity between behaviour and the prevailing social norms. Behaviour is not readily modifiable by adverse experience, including punishment. There is a low tolerance to frustration and a low threshold for discharge of aggression, including violence; there is a tendency to blame others, or to offer plausible rationalizations for the behaviour bringing the patient into conflict with society.

Personality (disorder):
· amoral
· antisocial

---

[46] ICD-10 website

· *asocial*
· *psychopathic*
· *sociopathic*

There is gross disparity between behaviour and the prevailing social norms[47]. Even where gambling one's life savings away in the middle of a desert is considered acceptable, to take so many drugs that a policeman's convention in Las Vegas appears to be entirely populated by lizards is significantly beyond the limits of "prevailing social norms". Looking back in history, would the normal man with a front row seat at the Mohammed Ali *Rumble in the Jungle* choose to float in a swimming pool with rotting marijuana instead of watch one of the greatest fights of the 20th Century? Paid a small fortune to cover a royal engagement, and flown 5000 miles to make the event, would a normal man decide to load up on cocaine and brandy and leave for home the very day he was meant to be on assignment?

In the UK, personality disorder is widely accepted as being untreatable[48]. Future legislation[49] makes provision for the preventative detention of the disordered in secure accommodation or prison. HST's type of potential diagnosis, particularly with

---

[47] Repeated deliberately

[48] It is treatable. Go to site below for details
http://www.dh.gov.uk/PublicationsAndStatistics/Publications/
PublicationsPolicyAndGuidance/PublicationsPolicyAndGuida
nceArticle/fs/en?CONTENT_ID=4009546&chk=BF%2B3ka

[49] The new Mental Health Bill to be written into Act at no certain date.

his fascination with firearms and violence, might not have been a free man if people stopped looking at the man as "ha! Crazy!" and started looking at him from the other criterion – "lock him up, quick!"

But this has wider implications. Might we consider Hunter S Thompson as a twenty-something year old who never grew up? A similar twenty-something year old to that whom parades naked on a porch, yelling abuse at police who about to break up the party he's at? A twenty year old who threatens to glass another woman for trying to sleep with the man she has targeted for wild sex later that night? The twenty-something year old who dresses up like a whore to take cocaine and drink hundred pound bottles of champagne in an R&B nightclub and lose all inhibition? The twenty five year old who takes cannabis and alcohol to get intoxicated until he gets paranoid schizophrenia and sticks a kitchen knife in a stranger's chest? Okay, not like Andrew. Andrew has paranoid schizophrenia which is a treatable mental illness!

This raises the wider question. If this behaviour is prevalent on a Friday night, then perhaps this is *"the prevailing social norm"*? It is certainly commented on by the media, not as a rare abstraction from the social norm because of isolated incident in a single city, but as a regular event across the United Kingdom. This behaviour is exploited and shown off on television programmes about Ibiza in summer, where British youth go for a cheaper experience of that found in the UK. From this perspective, of British people at home and abroad, Thompson follows the social norms so is not of the personality disorder by British standards.

The predominant behaviours are problematic. But they are behaviours sanctioned, even to the point of taxation by the authorities. Violent drunkenness and lewd behaviour is acceptable. Why then does society ask different questions of the man who smokes a drug that leaves him relaxed, tolerant and peaceable? The side effect of cannabis is paranoia, though is not directly linked to schizophrenia in the same way as alcohol is directly linked to liver cirrhosis[50]. The illness definitely caused by alcohol, liver failure, is acceptable whereas there is an unproved prevalence of an unacceptable illness among smokers of a drug that leaves them peaceful and introverted? George Best cheered to his grave and Pete Doherty hounded out of town.

The stigma of mental illness it seems, is promoted to fend off legalising drugs that make people peaceful and unlikely to participate in the violence and unacceptable behaviour that is the "social norm".

A suggestion? The crowd in Bristol city centre on Friday night show more psychiatric symptoms than does the crowd interned in Callington Rd

---

[50] See assertion in Dr Zammit's discussion in the chapter *Andrew*

mental hospital at the same time, the latter grouping of people being in medicated sleep. Which is a safer place, and of acceptable social norms on a Friday night at about midnight? Chatting unintelligible bollocks with someone under the watchful eye of a ward nurse, or shouting unintelligible bollocks, wary that that man could turn on you with the bottle in his hand, under the overstretched and brief gaze of a snatch team of police in the city centre? Do the police cancel all leave for a Friday night after the medication round in hospital, or do they do the same for the town centre on a Bristol City / Bristol Rovers derby day? Which crowd is more unpredictable? I prefer mental hospital, even Rampton, thanks!

To Hunter S Thompson, the diagnosis by an eminent doctor of his anonymous case can be boiled down to a simple sentence. We do not know what his illness was because he was blasted on drugs for the bulk of his adult life. The suggested treatment for Hunter S Thompson is a three to 6 month stabilisation or detoxification from narcotic intake. Only then could treatment be given for any underlying illness. Did he have any underlying illness? The answer is that until he had been detoxed, there is no answer. The final question, will we ever know? No, because of Thompson's suicide.

Suicide. People with illnesses that will leave them completely dependent on others and bereft of dignity might wish to kill themselves. A family friend of mine had to have her belly squeezed to defecate because her Multiple Sclerosis had taken away her ability to shit. She would have preferred to be remembered as a beautiful woman and wonderful mother, not a bag of shit that needed to be squeezed empty. (Jan died naturally unlike HST). Thompson apparently had no such illness. He even invited his son round, not to help his arthritic hands squeeze the trigger, but to watch his brains get spattered around his house. Is this a social act of a man of acceptable behaviour?

Mahalo

Junky

"Hi, my name's Richard and I am an alcoholic. Better, I am a dope fiend speed freak who's taken every drug under the sun, and no I haven't recovered – I have a cigar in my hand and I am pouring coffee down my neck at the rate of 2 pints an hour so I'm whizzing right now and best of all no Alcoholics or Narcotics Anonymous group can sensibly tell me to stop as they informally encourage it in initial abstinence!"

Robbie Williams is now famous for doing the same[51]. *The Sun* writes that he is in rehab for drugs that aren't generally considered dangerous, now he has stopped the traditional narcotics

---

[51] http://www.thesun.co.uk/article/0,,4-2007070393,00.html

GIVING VOICE TO THE INNER SCREAM

And daily he gets through an incredible 36 super-strength double espresso coffees, 60 Silk Cut cigarettes and around 20 cans of energy drink Red Bull.

In my speed freakery I am no original!

I have just been told to stop reading a book by Tam Stewart called *The Heroin Addicts*. The girlfriend told me to stop because even though I haven't had a drink for 23 months I am thinking like the addicted no hoper went off to do my MA before we met.

I start this chapter on addiction with my first of many insights – that a heroin addict is the same as an alcoholic, is the same as a benzodiazepine addict, the same as a nicotine addict. Nothing separates my boozing from the one in four adults who smoke a cigarette to wake up in the morning, or the guy who gets up at 6 in the morning to get to his dealer for a heroin fix. Addiction is not stigmatised like that, it gets at only the junky, whilst naming an airport after an alcoholic Irishman (another stereotype) who played football for 5 seasons at Manchester United.

Before we get down and dirty with the other types of addiction that are stigmatised, George Best was the alcoholic (who traded on his apparent ability to kick a ball when he was sober) who straightened me up. No, no fantastic light seen there, no halo around his head (other than the stink of whiskey). He had a drug called Antabuse implanted in his

stomach that, and he knew this, would kill him if he drank again. I
was under pressure to give up drinking for good at the same time, and hearing Best being given this was a new avenue for me to try. On the 3rd of March 2005 I was prescribed the drug.

Thank you, George Best. I am going to name the only accolade you really deserve. By dying you made me sober up. You aren't worth the piss on your deathbed for any other reason than, like Christ, you died to make the world a better place. For one man alone, so don't give me any shit about having an airport named after you, as that was named for the job you had that led to your alcoholism, and the praise I give you is for enabling me to sober up.

Addiction kills, and people remember people who die of it for that reason alone. My sister Julie. She was a great mother, and given practice on me as a child so our mother could work. Her daughter is now described as the Steve Irwin of Africa and her son, father to two and husband in Namibia, is doing well. Their mother? Died of liver failure.

Addicts are the same the world over. This chapter originally sought to distinguish the heroin addict from the rest of society for their illegal and much shamed addiction. I have changed course, I wish to relate us all as being the same, not that some are better than others. Needle in arm or cirrhotic liver, a dead addict is a dead addict. Also, that in life, an addict is an addict is an addict.

GIVING VOICE TO THE INNER SCREAM

I hoped to distinguish the pop star Pete Doherty from the once-football-player George Best, from the ex musician John Lennon, from the dead wife and mother Julie Hatton from her living brother Richard Shrubb from the nicotine addict Will Wilkinson. Can't. No sense in trying, in hackneyed addicts' words!

The chief reason for this diatribe? I was reading *The Heroin Addicts*[52] and my girlfriend saw me falling to pieces over the two weeks I was reading it. I would like to relate what messed me up when reading it. I'll try my best here.

Early Days

You talk a lot and have a feeling of wellbeing. It's a relaxation. The speedy effect turns into a deeper feeling later. When I'm on it I feel totally relaxed and feel nice. My problems all go away until I've got no gear again.[53]

Oh shit. I've run out of milk and need another coffee with my cigar while I am relating this to you. My problems have returned because I need my caffeine fix to stay in the zone and keep typing.

Or I might stay and tough it out. The old lady's off to Church and needs the air to be clean of cigar smoke for 2 hours before she goes as she's in the choir. Hold on, I am meant to be writing about

---

[52] Tam Stewart
[53] *The Heroin addicts* pp15

heroin addiction being the same as my particular fad of nicotine and caffeine…

Shooting up

Cranking is the most exciting, enjoyable and dangerous way to take heroin. It feeds the human capacity and need for ritual.[54].

Making tea.

Put the kettle on. Warm the teapot up before the water boils, placing the tea bag in after. Pour the hot water into the pot and let sit for 5 minutes. Pour, a third of a cup each until the cups are full. Add milk. It feeds the human capacity and need for ritual.

In my case, cut and light up an Alvarro Cedro and feel the hot smoke on the throat.

In seconds you could be lying there gaga with a bleached brain[55]

With too many cigars you could have a heart attack, the seriousness ranging from a tight chest to an embolism.

I knew heroin was supposed to be dangerous. People had warned me to stay away from it, but as I began to take it continuously and continued to feel fine I ceased to worry about it. I could not

---

[54] Ibid pp 21
[55] The Heroin addicts pp 21

understand what the fuss was all about. I felt great.[56]

I felt great. I was alone in the house, the adults burying my uncle Ivor. I had my sister's cider and cigarettes. I enjoyed every last moment of starting to die of nicotine addiction and joining my sister in her alcoholism. Life was great, I couldn't see the fuss. When Julie died in Africa on Feb 10th 2003 I wasn't interested in her death *from alcohol*, and was cast a hero because I tracked Mum down in an Andalusian hotel to pass on the terrible news. I commiserated with a drink, as I have been known to commiserate breaking a fingernail. I played the part of hard done by alcoholic afterwards to reap maximum social capital among fellow recovering alcoholics, telling them that I knew someone close who had died of it. Only, I wasn't telling them to help them recover, just telling them for something new to say to hide the fact I was cruising the path of recovery with no intention of recovering myself.

The cannabis connection

I cannot leave the question of how people come to embark on a career of heroin abuse without considering that old chestnut, the claim that cannabis plays a big part in leading onto the use of hard drugs.[57]

Personally? Everyone around me that was close thought that my abstention from alcohol was a

---

[56] Ibid pp35
[57] Ibid 39

greater plus than the minus of smoking dope. I was a happier stoner than a pisshead and people also liked me being stoned over being wired on coffee between alcohol binges. A gateway drug? Ask the politicians, who have now downgraded cannabis to the point kids don't get arrested for smoking it, whatever their age. I write in the previous chapter that there are more dangerous psychiatric symptoms in Bristol's city centre on a Saturday night than might be found in Rampton at the same time. I write here that there are more dangerous people addicted to God (George W Bush and Osama bin Laden). Drugs of any kind are known the world over to be good in moderation, I just wish I had had that lesson when I was 15 rather than now I am 32 and addicted to the speed–like rush of coffee and cigarettes…

What's it like being addicted to heroin?

The first thing you notice when you wake in the morning late, aching all over from sleeping too heavily and too long in one position… Then you remember. Realisation dawns. You need and you want drugs[58]

Realisation dawns, I need and I want drugs. Before I lift my head from the pillow to sip my coffee, I have a cigar in my mouth. The time in the morning differs because of my addiction, to coffee and nicotine, as opposed to heroin.

---

[58] Ibid 48

GIVING VOICE TO THE INNER SCREAM

… most addicts will recognise themselves in Pete's remark when he says, 'I've had a good go at the self pity business. I've given it the full bash…'

As have I. I was feeling really self piteous reading the text on which this chapter is based. I am a miserable addict, have been a miserable addict for the last 17 years. I just wish I hadn't discovered caffeine, nicotine, alcohol, LSD, speed…

The drug scene abounds with flippancy, wry humour and contradictory opinions, even from the same person. The life of a junkie is very much a life of highs and lows, a series of great swings between states of optimism and despair, between pleasure and pain.

Think of the world famous alcohol shooting gallery, *Cheers*. Or the *Rovers Return* or the *Queen Vic*. Three shooting galleries so central to communities of alcohol junkies that soap operas have been written about them. Soap operas, not documentaries because these aren't anything unusual, just such run of the mill life that from my standpoint, though I can watch a woman being stoned to death in a *Channel 4* documentary on Iran I find watching *Eastenders* so depressing I cannot bear it.

Everyone really wants a kilo. Then they can take it till the last gram and save that for an overdose. He was of course, joking but the underlying idea is clearly that no junkie would want to go on living once the smack ran out.

Conversation with psychiatrist in Weston Ward psychiatric unit in Bristol in 1999

"You can leave tonight if you want. What are you going to do once you leave hospital?

"I have two cases of beer and a bottle of whisky – what do you think?"

Doctor changes his mind and my coerced stay in mental hospital continued.

They eventually threw me out and I continued my merry way through heavy addiction where I could drink a pint of vodka and then had a quiet evening downing beer down the pub before coming home and blacking out on cider.

The addict goes through life wondering why no one understands him. People don't, not those on the outside of addiction. My greatest support on taking the early doses of Antabuse was not a fellow alcoholic in Falmouth but a woman just out of a US jail who had stopped her methamphetamine addiction. Kim was there for me at all hours by email. She knew every step I took, and understood every part of my recovery, *including* the years leading up to the day I quit for good.

Here's a picture, round which every addict in the world goes in recovery[59].

Figure 2, the Cycle of Change

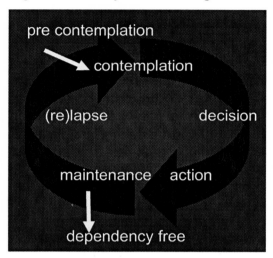

Here is the Cycle of Change. Round the merry way one travels, addicted to everything from sex to food to heroin. Going down to this level you're on a different spiral – you wake up, get your fix, get on with your day, fixing along the way, and then run out of money so get more. Spend that money and run out again…

---

[59] Figure 1 taken from www.alcohol-drugs.co.uk/themes/**Cycle**%20of%20**Change**.htm

To the diagram, at the so called rock bottom (though far from the earth's core or Hell) one starts on the Cycle of Change. Out of money or whatever other commodity one most needs be it friends or anything else, one contemplates giving up. One then makes the decision to give up.

"On the 1st January 2008 I will quit smoking" leads to the Action on the 1st, and for most smokers this lasts until the 3rd, through the phase known as Maintenance. On the 4th January you relapse and go through to Contemplation, whilst steadily going down the spiral of addiction. In the heroin user's case, this is stereotypically accompanied with a visit to the Magistrates and threat of a criminal record, or in George Best's case, a new liver…

So with a new liver, Georgey contemplated abstinence and maintained it for a few weeks. Sadly for him (and happily for me) the cycle stopped with his death, and I am dry 23 months later…

The cycle of change is the Merry-go-round round which all addicts must travel in recovery, be it heroin or cigarettes. In this knowledge, on failure of an attempt to stop smoking, I haven't even tried again for six months.

I played the system last time I was on the Cycle. Part of the conditions on which I would receive psychiatric treatment required that I detox from alcohol. Because I did not want to in my heart, I played games with them.

Not everyone wakes up to it. My sister didn't, nor did George Best.

In an interview with Professor of Psychopharmacology at Bristol University, David Nutt, he describes the way down:

There are four phases

1. *Fun. You get introduced to the drug and take it for pleasure*
2. *Fun goes away. At this stage you are taking it to avoid the rigours of daily living.*
3. *Dependence. In this way one forms a psychological need for the drug. This is different from the last phase, addiction, insofar as the body doesn't need the drug but the mind does.*
4. *Addiction. The body has made allowances and adapted to the drug, physical changes that only show their heads when the drug is withdrawn from the body.*

At the addicted phase, people will do anything to avoid the side effects of not having the drug on board. Professor Nutt suggests that the primary use of benzodiazepines by heroin and crack users is to soften the blow of withdrawal from the main drug.

The high is pedestrian by comparison to heroin and crack addiction; this is really only a way to avoid the symptoms of being strung out. There is a group of intravenous drug users in Glasgow however who are known to grind the benzos up and inject them in solution.

There are differences. Would I have drunk until I went yellow with jaundice as two people I have known did? Probably, because I had the same mantra as every addict on earth does …

It won't happen to me

It doesn't happen to the lung cancer sufferer on the TV advert. It didn't happen to George Best, nor did it happen to the last guy who mainlined a high dose of poisoned heroin and died with a needle in his arm…

So the addict decides to stop, and go through the *Cycle of Change* (see *figure 2*).

   1. Contemplation

"This is screwing my life up. I do not enjoy drinking fluids that make me gag for "fun" (in my case, spirits) and the holocaust is so old from my drinking that the clean up gang has been and gone after erasing my name from the memory of most of my so called friends."

People talk of a rock bottom at this stage. In truth I was looking so hard for the rock bottom I didn't see it for looking. I was happy in my shared house for loonies, I had raised it from a stigmatised loser in my own psychology to something that shouldn't be stigmatised, but rather, celebrated. I was having a whale of a time!

Rock bottom would finally gape at me, and I write in terms of an abyss rather than a place below which I could not go...

2. Decision

To stop.

The best decision in my own experience is not to stop after going down the pub tonight. The only time to stop is now, and that now has to extend to the end of today, and when I wake up that now is now and in the evening that now is now. Alcoholic's Anonymous state "One day at a time", and this is critical. I am 32. To state that I will still not have a drink age 80 is a high ambition, and to think of the shit I went through just to get out of the pit alcoholism dug for me, let alone the climb up the ladder I have afterwards, to say "I'll stop" beyond a day is ludicrous.

3. Maintenance

It ain't easy. Everything you ever did pissed / stoned / with a fag in hand, has to continue without that drug. Generally there is a watershed in your life as people realise just how great a guy you are sober, and people can be a real help. But not for long.

With the realisation that you're sober, people stop making the allowances they did for you when you were not. The hurdles are raised. Once more, if you lose your temper, or react negatively to anything that happens, people say to you "you're just like you were when you were drunk" and tell you to get lost. Whoaaa, I am the drunk who sobered up and I am a drunk again without drinking? Things escalate, and you need your relief again.

In this way, and through the pain one goes through in the physical stakes of sobering up, you have to really struggle. For instance no one told me about the mattress -soaking sweats that I would go through, a month after putting down my last drink. No one told me that after the major initial changes in my personality from the day I put down my last drink, that I would still be finding my way up a much gentler gradient two years later.

It is one of the major reasons I write this book; Mankind should understand before he or she judges. This is key to all human interaction, understanding *why* you will not give this person the time of day is key to reasoning that you *shall* not give that person that time of day.

There are many hurdles along the way. The stereotype of the shoplifting junky has one set of hurdles to go through regardless of whether he straightens up or not, the criminal record. This gives the authorities and all those who deal with you after you have given up, a paper memory of your antics while you were off your head. You have a criminal record that for at least 5 years you have to produce when you apply for a job. With the job market as competitive as it is, this makes it very difficult for someone to carry on being straight afterwards[60]...

The months following physical withdrawal are a crucial time. During that period, addicts need considerable support to re-orientate their lives if they are not to simply slip back into their old ways. Having a job to go to or some useful way of occupying your time is crucial to psychological welfare and, ultimately, to survival in a drug-free world. Addicts often say this, although in reality it is unlikely they will be offered a job...

John Wallace goes into some detail what a voluntary job does for his son with Cerebral Palsy and psychosis in the chapter, *Safety Net*. At the same time I write about stone cold sober people being refused work because they have an extra chromosome. A pale faced skinny junky...?

Providing someone with hope therefore, is key to recovery from drug addiction. This is where a variety of services come in. The Twelve Step programmes of Alcoholics' Anonymous, Narcotics'

---

[60] Stewart pp 166

Anonymous etc, provide a real chance for success.

One takes an aside here, to look at benzodiazepine addiction, a most middle class addiction insofar as the NHS doesn't recognise it in the way it regards heroin, so it is treated by the GP. Can't say whether Robbie Williams is / was on them... Andrew suggested he had taken them as a teenager with his booze[61]. You don't read newspaper reports of benzo addicts stealing toothbrush heads to sell for their next fix of Temazepam! Una Corbett, Director of the pressure group *Battle Against Tranquilisers (BAT)*, says that this is despite Valium, the most famous of the benzos being used as a unit of addiction

Martindale's Pharmacopeia measures all addiction against Valium, because it is the most addictive substance that exists!

This family of drugs has been prescribed since the 1960's to people with a range of mental health problems, and is prescribed to this day. They are also used for increasing the high one gets from alcohol and heroin; according to Una more than doubling the effect of the needle or drink one takes. A psychiatric medication with street value! They one of the hardest drugs to break free from, according to Una...

---

[61] See chapter *Andrew*

GIVING VOICE TO THE INNER SCREAM

"Coming off heroin was a piece of cake. Why didn't they tell me about benzos?" I was told this recently by a service user. The drugs are \a nightmare to come off – people become suicidal, have tinnitus, and the mental health problems the drugs are supposed to treat are often exacerbated by taking them. Service users will say that 98% of polydrug users will be addicted to benzos, the government states 89%. Clearly someone's wrong here and I doubt it is the service user.

Benzos are everywhere. I had a friend telling me that she was offered 50 diazepam for £90 down the pub the other day. This is a sign that they're getting harder to get hold of, drug dealers usually have them as a cheap secondary spend to the heroin and crack and sell them for between 50p and a £1 each.

There's been a crackdown on distribution of benzos lately. In 2004 the Chief Medical Officer wrote to all GP's, stating that they should only be prescribed for good reason. This reinforces a 1988 Committee for the Safety of Medicines ruling of the same thing, but this guidance was taken with a pinch of salt it seems, as the benzo problem never went away. What's happened this time is that many of the drugs have been classed as Controlled Substances under the Substance Misuse Act, and this imbues responsibility on the prescriber as to who gets them. They're still easy to get hold of – you can buy them on the Web for instance, and there are thefts from chemists, as well as private prescriptions. Even so, to handle private prescriptions, the government's done something quite clever, it now has a paper trail that leads between the drugs being issued and the doctor prescribing them, making it harder to remain anonymous when you prescribe them, you do illegally and you're in trouble in short.

+++++++++++++++

Professor David Nutt, of the Psychopharmacology Department of the University of Bristol, is sceptical of this. He says that this is largely because of media scare stories and government knee jerking in response.

+++++++++++++++++++
Una again

Another way people become addicted is through the inherited cases of doctors who have left their cases. A GP might move surgeries and their case is taken up by another, or the patient may leave one surgery and move on to another. In this way, people with these habits are given repeat prescriptions without monitoring.

These drugs are very nasty and people have been addicted to them for decades, I get people phoning up with a 35 year old habit of the drugs. Someone on them for that long is going to have a lot of difficulty coming off.

Homeless people? Getting these people off benzos is a nightmare. They buy them from their heroin dealers along with the other stuff, and then come into places like the Salvation Army hoping to get off all drugs, except that the Army won't detox them. Just too dangerous. In BAT's experience the best treatment for detoxing off benzos is in the community. It takes a while, and the service user must do it in the comfort of their home because it is so painful and takes a long time to come off. Thankfully the Army enables people to do their home detox there, so even for the destitute there is somewhere to round on this most difficult of addictions.

To put it in perspective, the advised benzodiazepine treatment programme for someone is four weeks, and the NHS recognises that this period must include a time for detoxing off the drugs even after that period. Yet people know how bad an addiction to this drug family is, so get extremely frustrated when they go in asking for a formal detox from street drugs, only to be turned away even by the Salvation Army because they're addicted to benzos. Not many understand the issue, some of these people are at a very hard rock bottom in their lives and face another round of rejection and re referral even by the people who are supposed to support them in their hour of need.[62]

The established way is now to get the homeless person a bed in a hostel, detox them off benzos and then get them a "detox bed" to clean them off the rest of the drugs. Having this problem, it really

---

[62] This is dealt with in the chapter, *The basket weavers and the basket case*

cuts down the amount of people who can get a detox bed at the Salvation Army, and everyone recognises it…. Well, almost everyone!

You see, the NHS denies that there's a problem. It recognises that there's a crack cocaine problem and that there's a heroin problem. It treats people with those problems through dedicated services. However, there is no formal route to come off benzos and GP's are held responsible for that detox programme. GP's have been prescribing these drugs for decades and face the real issues of taking people off them themselves. But no matter how they point this problem out, no one up the chain hears them.

+++++++++++++++

Professor Nutt is exemplary of powerful lobbying in this respect, the NHS not taking benzos too seriously. He is an eminent psychopharmacologist and feels that the benzo problem does not exist.

Now it's benzos. When will SSRI's (like Prozac and Seroxat) get the same treatment?

He was recently thrown off a government board of enquiry into Seroxat because he had shares in the company that patented the drug.

++++++++++++++++++

Back to Una

There's a study in the US which shows that 50% of alcoholics use benzos as well. This is understandable, given that the drugs affect the same neural receptors on the brain. Therefore you can put someone on Librium (one of the benzos), and take them off alcohol and it reduces the side effects of alcohol withdrawal. In this way you do a very sound and unproblematic use of benzos. The "Librium detox", as it is known, starts with a high dose of Librium, and the alcoholic stops drinking on that day, and the dose is rapidly reduced. It is very effective. People can have fits, sweats, the shakes… and all this is reduced with the Librium detox. Being a reducing dose, the user doesn't get addicted to the Librium and has a cushion on which to rest as he detoxes from the alcohol.

Other than this, with my experience, there is no other good reason to be put on them, and it is an awful experience coming off.

As this passage is written, so a spam email arrives saying that I can get Valium for $2.89 a pill[63]. Drugs of this kind are readily available on the internet and ultimately to drug dealers. If my faulty mouse told Google Autofill to put in my name, address and credit card details I could get the drugs without even thinking!

One needs to leaven the campaigner's angle with medical opinion. Professor David Nutt sees that there is no real reason for the user to become addicted to benzodiazepines for the simple reason that the high is not worth the while of the user…

---

[63] Go to this website to check!
http://calmorphan.com/legalrx/?page=valium&t=order&ref=&pid=2321&lang=&cart=

The bulk of polydrug users only buy these drugs when they cannot buy the quantity of the heroin they need. The drug takes the edge off their need, increasing the time they can last between fixes.

This is strongly opposed by Una, who responded by email saying the real reason for their use on the street...

Highs are not achieved with benzos on their own, but added to heroin or alcohol it more than doubles that effect!

Returning to the recovery from drugs in general, one looks to campaigning and community support organisations, a wide variety of which can be found in most cities. Turning to my personal experience again, I know at the base of removing an addiction, you have to want to stop.

Pressure from peers can go either way. Stewart writes of the community of junkies, and EJ Remes did a study of masculinity and drug addiction. She hypothesised that because of masculine traits men go the extra mile of heroin addiction. Initial observation of the community at the Salvation Army hostel suggested heroin is a rite of passage for some groups of young men[64].

Drinking to excess and taking other drugs, speeding in cars and being involved in criminal

---

[64] EJ Remes (2004) *Masculinity, risk taking behaviour and injecting drug use* Unpublished paper

activities are all attributed to the behaviours of young men and are considered to be a test of boundaries of fear and endurance, and attempt to prove adulthood or masculinity

I draw a parallel with my time prior to my MA. The pub was fun and getting blasted a real pleasure. Thursday night for my group of friends in Bristol, payday from the DSS triggering it. Going to college was the same at first, until my 30th birthday in November 2004.

The class had sung Happy Birthday and then agreed to meet down a soulless Wetherspoons for drinks afterwards. I obliged after 2 bottles of Rioja to join them and did not buy a drink all night. The squalor of the memory ranks large in my mind. What did I do for my 30th birthday? Got pissed with a load of Mummy subsidised twenty-something's. What did I do the Friday before? Got pissed with a load of Mummy subsidised twenty-somethings... I think the difference was that the night was marginally cheaper than most nights. Remembering the Hollywood film, *Groundhog Day* each time I went out on the piss, I was not to sober up for 4 more months…

Remes identifies two personalities that she found in the men she studied for her Social Work MA thesis[65]

---

[65] Remes (2004) Unpublished

The first image was exposed during key-work sessions or private conversations, and was based upon emotionally damaged personalities in which they related their difficulties within life back to an early age. During these sessions the men would usually identify emotions of powerlessness, weakness and worthlessness. The second image, that was also inherent to the environment of the hostel, was an image of macho behaviour. I found that this behaviour could be identified at its greatest when the men were situated in groups and pretences of being tough, brave, violent and risky would subsequently emerge.

This dichotomy is prevalent in nearly every addict. The "addict persona" is brave, tough and hard. He enjoys the thrill of the score, the taking of the drug and he is king of the world when he is off his face. Saturday night down the town centre – the old proverb, "laugh and the whole world laughs with you, cry and cry alone" comes to the fore. Getting pissed on a Saturday night and having a whale of a time is de rigueur for the growing and successful twenty-something. The most successful man down the pub, to the measure of that environment, is the one who is pissed up and waltzes over to the long legged babe in a short skirt and whirls her off her feet before taking her home and ravishing her for after-hours entertainment. He certainly doesn't go over to her to talk about his feelings about the world that has wronged him! Another place to be big and hard is the bike sheds at school as the "hardest" kids inhale their first cigarettes...

GIVING VOICE TO THE INNER SCREAM

But equally in the headspace of the late stage addict is a feeling of loss and hopelessness, as described above. Stewart describes the heroin addicted man as being a great lover at first, an all night shag, before his addiction makes sex of little interest...

It is, literally, quite true that under heroin's influence people can make love more or less all night...[66]

In the end, sex, like eating, loses its attraction for junkies. They simply run out of libido...[67]

As I write I hear on the radio that Boots the chemist is about to sell Viagra over the counter in Manchester. A hedonist vox popped for the radio described using it as being a great way to have a night out and then manage to get it up afterwards, ending the famous "Brewer's Droop" problem with a little blue pill. The hedonist can now be a man from the first pint to the last vinegar stroke in the wee hours.

But the masculinity soon loses its potency. I enjoyed the manliness of addiction to alcohol, but in a new environment I found that it didn't appeal. Besides, the last time I pulled after a 10 pinter was in my early twenties! You grow up, I suppose. I went from being a rebel with a cause at school, and became a hedonist at sea and into my twenties whilst watching it all go wrong around

[66] Stewart pp41
[67] Stewart pp 43

me. Seeing it all go wrong made me more inclined to share my problems and outlook on the world with a good lady friend than stick my hot rod between her legs, this is apart from the fact that my hot rod was hardly glowing and rigid!

I am lucky that no one prescribed benzodiazepines for anxiety. Una Corbett says that anxious people can become addicted to benzos,

Benzos cause anxiety after a while. After a period of taking them you get more anxious and need more. This is due to the body developing tolerance for the drugs and needing more to sate. It is also because a side effect of taking them is it causes anxiety, in the same way as another psychiatric medication may cause involuntary twitching.

Professor Nutt disagrees

People who end up on benzos for anxiety are just anxious people. That they've been on benzos for 35 years is purely because they've been anxious for that period

Both cite scientific articles. Una sees the victims of benzo addiction because she is a leading light in campaigning against, and treating it. She is biased though, and Professor Nutt the opposite way. I leave it for the reader to judge.

To my alcohol addiction, I was lost in a world of anxiety and not being able to understand why people avoided me outside the alcohol and psychosis worlds. In many ways my masculine side rotted away, leaving someone so desperate to reach out to someone, that I had become effeminised.

The cure in the end was a combination of drug therapy for alcoholism and getting my head straight, and conjoining the two personas of addict and "lost, emotionally damaged man". It was this coalescence that straightened me out in the end.

I guess it was George Best that enabled the coalescence and convalescence to take place, it appealed to my masculine side that I would die if I drank again. "I will die if I drink and I don't want to die" appealed more than "I will get diarrhoea if I drink this" (I had the shits each time I drank). It was something to brag about too, "don't buy me alcohol or I'll be in hospital" was a great way to put it across, over "I have quit drinking, not for me thanks" (which had never worked).

Ending my relationships with fellow drinkers helped too. One of the biggest things a junky must do is break contact with his fellow users. People are in a community, and that community is essential for at its most basic we are a social animal. I refer again to the shooting galleries of *The Rovers Return* and the *Queen Vic*. In the end a world where no one had known me beyond a few months and which left me under no illusion that weirdness was forbidden in their world, shook me into the unalterable truth, that if I was to rejoin society I must quit drink.

I was in a social hole, and in the process had developed a relationship with two women on the course that I did not see a problem with, but they did. I knew they did because the Dean of Faculty pulled me up about it. In part because they wanted a dangerous liaison with a schizophrenic, and in part because I gave them more of it than they could chew, I was eventually hauled up for it and threatened with being thrown off the course for effectively stalking them.

On the 3rd March 2005 I went to see my psychiatrist. I put him under pressure, and truthfully said that I would prefer to be psychotic as a side effect of Antabuse (the main reason I was denied the drug at the Robert Smith Unit in Clifton). He agreed and 23 months on I sit here finishing a chapter of a book. I am well, no more the schizophrenic with whom a dangerous liaison is possible for the simple reason that I do not present myself as strange in any way. My girlfriend sees me as a pillar of strength, and I often question this because I do not always see the man she does. Even Dena and Kirsty saw this man, as exhibited in a hug and a farewell kiss at the class booze cruise at the end of the course.

I am still that man though, as much the addict as the practising alcoholic or the junky who stole some toothbrush heads at the supermarket this morning and is relaxed and amenable now. Why?

GIVING VOICE TO THE INNER SCREAM

I'll put my keyboard down to get a coffee and a cigar now!

The basket weavers and the basket case

"Get a job you bum".

"I don't buy the *Big Issue* – its begging"

"Junky loser"

Three commonly used phrases in regards the homeless. People view this group as weak and who generally have themselves to blame for their housing situation. What then of the two former inmates of Rampton and Broadmoor who have nowhere to sleep and turn up at Bristol's Salvation Army hostel periodically? They have nowhere else to go and have been dumped by a system that in another chapter of this book seems so keen to keep them stable and free from relapse. What of the "Schedule 1 offenders" who get hounded from any home they have because of previous sexual offences against children and are forced to roam the streets? What of the man who becomes homeless not of a wish to be free from responsibility, but whose personal priorities become warped by the drug he's addicted to?

These people in most cases have somewhere to sleep after a recent government drive to re-house the homeless. The government initiative only went so far however, and after the well publicised campaign to get the homeless off the streets, did little more to achieve the next step, getting them out of temporary accommodation and into a fixed place of residence[68].

To be homeless and mentally ill is of high chance, there is over a 50% prevalence of mental illness amongst homeless young people as a 2006 Centrepoint study showed[69]:

It seems reasonable that in most cases the loss of one's home will bring about stressors that can deplete an individual's mental health. Thus, it is estimated that between 30% and 50% of single people experiencing homelessness have mental health problems compared with between 10% and 25% of the general population (Warnes et al 2003). More specifically in a London based study of young people experiencing homelessness in which psychiatric diagnostic criteria were used, two
thirds met the threshold for a mental disorder. In the same study 70% of those with a diagnosable mental illness had experienced their first symptoms before their first episode of homelessness.

---

[68] National Statistics say that the amount of people trebled in London in the five years to 2002. See the website http://www.statistics.gov.uk/cci/nugget.asp?id=386

[69] Centrepoint (2006) *Making the link between mental health and youth homelessness, a pan – London study* Mental Health Foundation

It seems likely that as well as creating or exacerbating mental health problems, homelessness might itself be precipitated by a mental illness. There is also the possibility that other factors may put individuals at risk of both homelessness and mental health problems. Against this backdrop Centrepoint (2005) has reported a lack of adequate provision to manage the increase in mental health problems amongst young people, which if untreated can lead to far greater long-term problems. People who live in bed and breakfast or hostels are 8 times more likely than the general population to experience mental health problems, and those who sleep rough are at 11 times the risk ...

It stands to reason that facing homeless is pretty depressing, and the very route to being mentally ill incurs not a little poor thinking and strategising; your brain is being rewired the wrong way after all. Whether the chicken or the egg in terms of homelessness being the reason or the result of mental illness, there is a high prevalence of mental illness in this sector.

Add to this, drug problems. There is a high prevalence of drug problems among the homeless. Indeed part of the stereotype of the jobless bum is one who drinks or jacks up all the money he gets. Centrepoint discusses this[70]...

---

[70] Ibid 69

GIVING VOICE TO THE INNER SCREAM

The relationship between substance use and homelessness is complex and can be reciprocal in nature. Thus, substance use may lead to a period of homelessness, which in turn may worsen the substance use behaviours. In a study of young people experiencing homelessness across England and Wales 73% were found to be current drug users, a majority of whom had left home because of family conflict. However, of those who were using heroin and/or cocaine more than half started only after becoming homeless. Similarly, in a pan-London study of homelessness among all age groups 83% were found to be substance users and their levels of dependency and the likelihood of them injecting drugs increased the longer they remained homeless.

There are a variety of problems faced once the person is made homeless and seeks help. The chief reason I started this chapter was on hearing of a Catch – 22 faced by the homeless mentally ill. Accessing primary care (such as a GP) is difficult because you generally have to have a home mailing address for a surgery to take you on its books, yet you generally have serious medical problems. As time went on, the investigation changed for a far worse problem. Many people turning up to shelters and hostels have mental health and drug needs, so the organisations on the front line must refer them to secondary mental health services. These in turn make it difficult because they are some of the most difficult patients and statutory services either just don't want to help, or pass them on between various sectors of the system. Between the drugs rehabilitation and the mental health system for instance.

Who picks up the pieces when they are scattered beneath the net? The Voluntary Sector is a good place to start, organisations that supplement the government where the government fails or has no wish to act on their behalf. An article on the Centrepoint website in 2006 stated[71]

... despite these figures staff working within housing and youth homelessness services lack the necessary skills to deal with mental health issues and need specialist training. They also struggle to access appropriate support for young people experiencing mental distress. Mental health assessment waiting times are long and this lack of early intervention leaves young people vulnerable to developing more entrenched mental health problems. As a result young people often reach crisis point before being seen by a mental health team.

... some voluntary sector housing and homelessness support services encounter barriers when trying to refer young people to the statutory sector. This is because mental health services are under resourced and some statutory services are reluctant to accept referrals from the voluntary sector. The research also found that young people with both mental health and drug and alcohol

---

[71] Full article available at
http://www.centrepoint.org.uk/content/view/183/41/

problems often do not get the help they need because services rarely work together making it difficult to provide complete care packages.

"*Some statutory services are reluctant to accept referrals from the voluntary sector.*"[72] In many cases people turn up at hostels' doors in a rather fragile frame of mind; you might imagine that on the day you were evicted you would be! As I will describe later on in the chapter, statutory services in Bristol are often referred people that they deem unnecessary to be referred and a certain amount of thinning must be done among the distressed down to the "Seriously Mentally Ill".

In an email interview Dr Jan Melchiar, Consultant Psychiatrist at the Bristol Specialist Drugs Service (BSDS) avers that at least one community mental health team (CMHT) in Bristol takes on no one with depression;

...the CMHTs have very varying criteria about what is a mental illness that they will take on, which is dependent on many issues. The biggest is lack of resource. For example, elsewhere in the past, due to chronic staffing shortages, one CMHT decided not to accept any patient for treatment who was suffering from depression.

This has caused some tension between the voluntary sector and the community mental health

---

[72] Repeated deliberately

teams in Bristol, as will be shown later. The Salvation Army is almost shorthand for what one needs to do in such a situation – similar to what you do if you're stuck at a train station up north, you head for Crewe - if you're homeless you go to the Sally Army for help. So I did, and went to find out about their problems in getting people help.

The hostel in Little George Street in the centre of Bristol does not meet the stereotype of the homeless hostel. It is not 1930's housing stock, nor is it 1950's grey and industrial. Rather, a 1990's era, warm and clean tower block that sits near to the large building site of what will be the extended Broadmead shopping centre.

For a management perspective on the hostel, I spoke to its Centre Manager, Anne Babb.

The Salvation Army Hostel is a 93 bed, men only hostel. There are 69 beds for the homeless who may walk through the door at any time. Additionally we have 24 detoxification beds, for drug detox preparation, detox and rehabilitation.

The Salvation Army hostel in Bristol is foremost among its peers, we can get people healthcare and secondary treatment quickly and effectively. Our talisman in that
respect is our Social Worker Margaret Mitchell, who works on site. Having her means the mental health and other services take us seriously because of her qualifications and reputation in the city. Other hostels aren't so lucky, they do not

generally have the expertise on site to look at a case and give potential diagnoses or suggested treatment programmes for the people who turn up at their doors.

They get someone behaving strangely through the door and they say "nutter, needs help". We however can look at his background and say "possible diagnosis of psychosis…" and pass on to the exact authority that can help. If we didn't, like some hostels there would be problems in communication with the authorities and time wasted on both counts. In this way Margaret saves us and the Statutory Sector time with her expertise.

As such we do not have the problem you cited in your approach to me. It is not a bed of roses. Though professionals in Bristol take our suggestions seriously, it is a constant battle to get treatment for our clients whether it is for drugs, mental health or even simple primary care.

One of our hardest battles is over dual diagnosis, polydrug users. In plain English, this means people who have mental health problems and a drug habit that consists of two or more narcotics. The current trend is for speedball addiction, people addicted to taking crack cocaine and heroin simultaneously either by smoking or intravenously. Much more insidious however is their addiction to benzodiazepines. These people have been prescribed things like diazepam for mental health problems and because they are so addictive and provide a nice high in quantity, buy it illegally or get illicit prescriptions (via theft, manipulation of GPs…) Because they're prescribed the drugs for mental health problems we cannot give them a detox bed, because those beds are for people to get completely clean and it might be dangerous for our staff if we detoxed them from benzos to uncover a dangerous streak of mental illness.

Our detox beds are well staffed and a comfortable place to get over the rigours of hard drug addiction. However in order to deal with someone with a benzo addiction we would have to be better staffed. You, Richard, have said you won't come off your neuroleptic medication because you don't know what would happen to you if you did. If you came in we could clean you up off all the other drugs and keep you on your olanzipine. But benzos are taken medicinally as well as recreationally, and the mix means we'd have to take you off the benzos as well.

As such we have to approach the Primary Care Trust to bring them off the benzos and get them referred to the CMHT for their mental health problems before we detox them. You'd think this a simple thing to do – get them treated for their mental health, get them detoxed from benzos and then get them a detox bed. In an ideal world this would be so! However with the two authorities, the drug rehab and the mental health, they pass clients between them willy nilly. Thus the mental health case will be passed from the drugs project

to the mental health system without treatment and the mental health system will insist that the BSDS detox them because they cannot see the mental health problem until they're detoxed.
++++++++++++++++++++

In the preceding chapter, I spoke to Una Corbett from Battle Against Tranquilisers about this drug family, and for balance to an expert in psychiatric medication. In another chapter I look at Hunter S Thompson, and referred his case to a psychiatrist. His response was *we cannot diagnose his symptoms as a mental health problem until he is clean of all the illegal narcotics he has taken*[73]. In the first chapter Dr Zammit explains that drug use can simulate psychiatric symptoms, indeed that some drugs are used in laboratory tests to induce the symptoms for study of the brain[74].

As such this uncaring game of pass the parcel is symptomatic of retrenched psychiatric doctrine based on scientific fact, you cannot treat a man for paranoia if that paranoia will stop after he has recovered from cannabis use. When asked for a second angle to HST, Dr Melchiar says that they aim for stability in the patient before treatment for the psychiatric issues.

Stability allows the patient to have the time and space to start to address their problems. In the case of most people we treat who are, admittedly, at the 'difficult-to-treat' end of the spectrum,

---

[73] See Hunter S Thompson chapter
[74] See the chapter on Andrew

stability may initially involve time on a stable dose of replacement medication e.g. methadone or buprenorphine. After all, if someone has had 10 years to learn that the solution to all problems is to take illicit drugs such as heroin, they require more than a quick detox to develop new ways of dealing with life's problems.

Similarly, common sense prevents the drugs services from detoxing a man from psychiatric medication. You take the writer off his schizophrenia medication and he would not be a writer but a pirate radio DJ with a listener of one. You take the "psycho killer" Andrew, off his antipsychotic medication and he doesn't want to know what would happen.

An October 2006 Masters thesis quotes a homeless man in such a situation[75]:

I've had dual diagnosis so every service has bounced me back saying… mental health team said that (name of service omitted) had to see you and (name of service omitted) say that mental health have to see you, so in the end I have given up basically. I have had no service or no help from both of them. Because of this dual-diagnosis… I found it like being bounced back like a tennis ball"

---

[75] Gregoriou, A (2006) *Service user perspectives in dual-diagnosis: and study on dual-diagnosis within homelessness services for men of between 18-59 years* Unpublished pp 31

GIVING VOICE TO THE INNER SCREAM

These men aren't tennis balls! They are of the most vulnerable adult group in society and are crying out for help from any and every service that they can, yet for a variety of supposedly rational reasons about safety and clinical doctrine, they give up all hope of help and live in fear that their drugs habits and mental health problems do not result in extremely serious consequences.

To Dr Melchiar again:

Funding. You cannot have joined up thinking and a proper flow of dual diagnosis if there is no funding for it. Currently, there is very little funding for it. In Bristol, for example … there are over 20 Mental Health teams who could, potentially, be involved with our patients. All of them are under pressure, financially, with posts either unfilled or frozen, due to fiscal needs. Trying to add to this by having joined-up thinking without any funding for it is difficult.

Lynette Duff of the Inner City Mental Health Team says later on in this chapter that AWP is in motion to remedy the joined up thinking approach Dr Melchiar complains about. As time progresses, the situation might just improve…?

We return to Anne Babb on what the Salvation Army does for its clients.

The hostel staff's biggest job is advocating on behalf of the dual diagnosis homeless on individual cases. In the system, persistence in our experience pays dividends, pushing and badgering the statutory services into providing support and care for these men achieves results. Why do we need to do this on a daily basis? For the last six years we have had a consistent stream of dual diagnosis homeless men, approximately 90% of the people who come through our doors have these problems. By now you'd have thought that there would be a system in place to get someone treatment for their illnesses.

The Inner City Mental Health Team (ICMHT) in Bristol had a solution, a Community Psychiatric Nurse (CPN) for the homeless, which is a post paid for by the Avon and Wiltshire Partnership mental health NHS Trust (AWP). Consequently we had someone at the other end of the phone who realised that these men had dual diagnosis and would provide a first statutory step into the psychiatric system. She was good at her job and our job was made easier, particularly so with Margaret Mitchell being another professional in the same field to have eye to eye conversations about the cases that she was referring on. In this way the system worked, to the point that when the Office of the Deputy Prime Minister withdrew the original funding for the post, AWP kept the post on from its own funding. The proof is in the negative, she has been off work for some time and communication with the ICMHT is almost as difficult as it was before the post was started.

Add to this, the benzos cases. The NHS doesn't recognise the problem in the same way as they do say, drug and alcohol addiction. Thus though there is a treatment programme in place for heroin and speedball addicts there is no formal structure in place to treat benzo addicts. This is despite the NHS in its various forms prescribing the drugs to people for a variety of mental health problems, especially to those people who are of itinerant address, for panic attacks, depression and other times where the patient is overwrought due to his situation. The patients like their prescription because they can take a large dose and be relieved from the emotional pain that ails them, or load up on them for the fun of it.

A situation of a pot calling the kettle black here? Because the Salvation Army cannot look after them they pass them to the BSDS who pass them to the CMHT (who pass them back). However the SA do not dump them on the street in the same way as the NHS does; indeed, it lets them live there and actively fights on their behalf to get the right treatment decided upon and given.

But what of the problems on the front line? Margaret Mitchell is the Salvation Army hostel's Social Worker. She is employed so that they have a stronger idea of whom to refer, and where to refer them, for treatment in the statutory sector. It is her job to assess new clients, and get them the treatment that they need. Anne Babb feels that she is a big reason that the health system will talk to the Salvation Army over other hostels which might not have someone of the same qualification. Being able to talk to the authorities on their terms is essential if one is to get the treatment people need.

Margaret describes the people that turn up at the hostel's door.

Up to about six years ago we had a population of clients who were mostly burned out alcoholics and schizophrenics, men of the road for the most part who went from city to city to do casual labour and to drink their earnings. From about 2001 however the demography changed here, for some reason we started to get a lot of homeless dual diagnosis heroin addicts, and over the years this has in turn changed to the point that 90% of our clients are now young white males addicted to heroin and crack cocaine as well as having mental health problems.

These people are banned by law and the Christian ethos of the church from taking their drugs on site, but they are practising addicts with generally very serious mental health problems. Many have moved cities to disappear and commit suicide; you Richard said you have known one such man who was re-housed in supported housing. You tell me he is settled in a council flat which is modified to his physical disability (though he had alcohol problems and no history of hard drugs).

When they arrive here they are generally frightened and confused, and want a roof over their head. They generally have no contact with the statutory services, and are glad to be offered accommodation. There are various ethnicities of people who walk through our doors, they might be of another country but generally they are from Bristol.

We cannot always offer them somewhere to sleep, we are generally at 95 - 98% capacity. This means we have to prioritise the beds for the most needy and find somewhere else for the people we cannot house.

They're at different places on the cycle of change[76]. This means they're not always trying to stop, though equally so some have a strong wish to. Those people that do are provided with one of the detox preparation beds we have here. Off heroin and completely on replacement therapy, they will pass up the line to the Subutex detox beds and hopefully then onto the rehabilitation unit.

Their lives are always chaotic. Dominated by drugs and hindered by their mental health problems, life is a real struggle. A large number have "Hospital Orders"[77] which mean that they have been in secure psychiatric units. There are two homeless people in this area who have been recently freed from Broadmoor and Rampton with no follow up care, supervision or treatment; they're dangerous and need help in order to be safe from themselves and others. Another was banned from

---

[76] See this in chapter, *Junky*

[77] Are being watched under Section 117 of the 1983 Mental Health Act, but not detained.

the county of Cornwall because he took his family under siege, threatening to kill them with a shotgun. The public can relax because we got him a bed in the local Regional Secure Unit!

There is a pattern of admission and readmission to mental hospital. They are on the streets until they are "deemed of danger to themselves or others" under the 1983 Mental Health Act when they are taken off the streets and Sectioned. They are kept in for the duration of their Section and then released into the community with little or no follow up care. They become ill again, find themselves on the streets, and the cycle turns again.

There is a scheme called Supporting People[78] *which is a government grant system to ensure that people get tenancy support and ultimately do not wind up homeless. Yet if he does not pay his rent because he has spent it on drugs, he will wind up homeless.*

Add to this one of society's most stigmatised groups, the so called Schedule One *offenders, paedophiles and child abusers. What qualifications are we supposed to have? Probation Officer, Social Worker, CPN... I keep a log of who and what might be found in the hostel, whom to watch for and whom to care for. We see mental health problems in the same light as a Middle Englander would a broken leg, but some of the*

---

[78] See this in *Supporting People* chapter

most dangerous and unpredictable people in society come here for relief.

There is a subgroup of people who come here to change their identity for a variety of reasons, yes, like the legend of the French Foreign Legion. You can imagine why, though it makes life easier and safer for us if we can get a handle on what their background is. There was a man who self referred recently, and had changed his name. I didn't think he was well and within half a day I found out exactly what the problem was; he had escaped a London Regional Secure Unit and had a history of violence toward women. The authorities were jumping up and down over this, since the last thing he'd done was knock on Number 10 Downing Street's door to ask Tony Blair for a £5er!

Then there are the power struggles. Bristol City Council has a stranglehold on the mentally ill homeless. It is fine fighting so jealously for control of a subgroup of people but in amongst the infighting, a psychotic person is still psychotic. While people are deciding whom should treat someone and how, they still need treatment.

From this, one will aver that the situation for the homeless seriously mentally ill is a basket case in its own right. It appears to show thought disorder and apparently makes strange decisions as to how to deal with the client. It shows psychosis insofar as not making the rational decision of how to treat someone. Dealing with this mess are the likes of the Salvation Army, who are responsible for looking after the parts of society that no one else wants to treat; paedophiles, dangerous mentally ill and drug addicts. So much for the "cradle to grave policy" of the Welfare State!

Or not. The reason the Salvation Army benefits from having Margaret Mitchell on site is that she is a first sieve of the seriously-screwed-up-about-being-made-homeless-this-morning, and the "Seriously Mentally Ill". She is qualified and experienced in telling who should be treated and who should not be. Tensions arise with the statutory services when they take the group she refers on, and whittle this down still further.

In a sometimes taught and difficult interview putting the Salvation Army's case to her, I interviewed Lynette Duff, manager of the Inner City Mental Health Team in Bristol, about the provision of mental health services to the homeless. Due to the tension that arose in the interview, what follows is the transcript, and not the edited highlights of the interview as elsewhere in the book...

Richard - Why do homeless people find it difficult accessing healthcare?

Lynette - *I think that's an interesting question. That is the perspective of the voluntary sector. We as a team have looked at this. Primarily it is because there is a lack of understanding of serious mental illness and a lack of training in the voluntary sector, possibly there's a lack of clarity as to how to access the service. This is though we have had a single point of entry for the last three years now. As part of the development of services we now have one number as a point of contact. I guess it is like the question about AWP losing staff and people quoting it is really difficult getting service from secondary mental health service. From our perspective this is not the case, but that is... it depends on who you speak to.*

Maybe we're not clear enough as to what our criteria are for admission because we are a secondary mental health service, and are for people with serious mental health problems who I hope are able to access the service. For the last couple of years and certainly since May we've had the Assessment and Intervention Team which we've widely circulated with leaflets and information so the voluntary sector can refer straight into, and there's a phone number to access the service you need. So I think historically it has been difficult to access the service but now it is not the case.

Could we talk a bit about the Community Assessment and Intervention Team (CAIT team). Could you tell me how it works, what it is... ?

The Assessment and Intervention service for the central sector, and it offers short term intervention for people up to three months currently. The whole philosophy behind that was that bringing people into the service, they received support and a new experience, very much taking on the recovery models, which is about giving people hope and looking at people in terms of episodes of care and looking at people's strengths and being quite clear about the type of service we're providing and why, what the expectations are from both the service users perspective and what we can realistically offer and that is open to all homelessness agencies who do refer. I could look at the stats and we are getting increasing numbers of referrals.

So, what sort of numbers. Do you have them to hand?

I could get them, we are getting increasing numbers. We are getting referrals from various agencies that are in contact with Phil Willshire who's our team manager of the Assessment and Intervention Team. We've also recently recruited a Somalian mental health worker who deals with a group who are often homeless and not as obvious as the street sleepers who may be sleeping on people's sofas, or wherever and aren't... It is important to cover this group and as such we have recruited him.

Through the CAIT team, what seems to be the major problem... you seem to say that there isn't one. What sort of problems have you observed... in respect of self referral or voluntary sectors referring to you?

As far as I am aware and with reference to the CAIT team we have seriously improved our service but it was always an option and I think it is a lack of communication, a lack of understanding around how to access services. Now I think we have to hold our hand up and accept some responsibility for that and I think certainly since I have been here, we have been reviewing our service with a view to improving access, which is part of the drive from government and the Trust. So there… if there is a problem with referrals people are not feeding that directly back to us. So if people aren't telling us they are having problems referring to us, then we can't really …

So I think it's interesting you said you've interviewed Margaret Mitchell and two other people?

I've interviewed Margaret Mitchell and her boss Anne Babb who both sort of raised this issue, I went in under the impression that is was primary healthcare that people had difficulty getting, therefore getting access up the chain, but they were saying that certainly in their case, they were saying that the Salvation Army certainly have an Approved Social Worker there who works, who can make an assessment of site, and who can give you a clear understanding of the situation that Joe Bloggs might be in and the process will be a lot smoother than say another homeless hostel without a social worker on site.

I wasn't aware that the Salvation Army had an Approved Social Worker on site because they have to be employed by the council so I'm not sure…

Sorry she's qualified as an Approved Social Worker

She's not an Approved Social Worker and I know that because she was a student in the team I was a Social Worker in!

She's always worked in the Salvation Army since she's qualified. So she isn't an Approved Social Worker and I think it's really important and it's an opportunity to debunk some of the myths that are around and you can quote anecdotal stuff from Margaret Mitchell but she's one small part of the picture and she doesn't have a lot of contact with us actually.

Sorry… I didn't know the difference… my fault. Wasn't told whether she was Approved or not…

The Salvation Army, and I think we've got the stats broken down and I'll give them before you go, and you know refers to us, and um Margaret has some knowledge and obviously she's very experienced in working with homelessness, I think there's a lot of.. err…, I don't know how to describe it, I think it is about making sure we communicate effectively, and what we pass on as fact, rather than ahh, making judgements and assumptions. There have always been tensions between the voluntary sector and secondary mental health services, and in a way I think that's right – there should be, I think, however in my experience a lot of what is said by some of the voluntary sector, we have to hold our hand up and say I think resources have been always an issue, but in terms of access to the service we have always had a clear route of access and people are responded to right away IF they meet our criteria and I think that's where the tension sits. It maybe that the Salvation Army feel this person has a serious mental illness but when we go and assess them with a very experienced team of people, in our view they do not need secondary mental health services and should be seen and followed up in primary care, and actually there are very limited primary care services which adds to the problem so everything comes to the secondary services. And if we think of the whole stigma in terms of bringing people into secondary services unnecessarily, its massive and I think we have an underdeveloped primary care mental health service because obviously they want to get people the right support and help, turn to secondary services and obviously we're not an unlimited resource. I think that's where the tension sits.

[The stats she referred to are still not on my desk. One will assume she's right…]

Okay, so… I came into the system 7 years ago. I had no problems getting into the system with full blown paranoid schizophrenia. What constitutes a serious mental illness that doesn't constitute … What constitutes a mental illness that should be treated with primary care?

We follow the Building Bridges guideline and what falls within that definition. Building Bridges was one of the first documents and currently the Trust is reviewing their entry and exit criteria. For access to social services people have to meet the Fair Access to Care Criteria, so we do follow very closely guidelines that, in terms of access to the system. Because generally people without psychosis, people who are treated with depression, are usually managed in primary care. It depends on the complexity, I mean overall if people are so depressed their social circumstances begin to break down, obviously that level of depression is serious enough to warrant an intervention. I must stress we're not a "psychosis only service" and of course that includes people who are homeless.

And actually our home intervention team has worked with people in the Salvation Army. They get a home intervention service in the hostel. We do not discriminate against people who are homeless.

One of the things they raised, and I have found out from elsewhere too, I tried to get a dead writer diagnosed. He'd been taking drugs all his life, and the response from the academic psychiatrist was to detox him first and this seems to be a problem people face throughout the system, is that they've got a benzodiazepine and a speedball addiction but they've also got a mental illness. The Salvation Army seems to have difficulty referring to the mental health teams because they seem to say "clean them off the drugs", they go to the drug teams, and the drug teams say "clear them from their mental illness first". What's your response to this?

I think the information you're getting (haha) from the Salvation Army is very biased and one sided, which, is fine, and thank you for giving me the opportunity to put our perspective because almost all our service users in the Inner City team have a dual diagnosis. There is no way we tell people to get detoxed and cleaned up. What we are doing is trying to develop much closer working relationships with the BSDS and we've got a meeting I think the week after next for instance to look at how, because what we would like is part of the CAIT team. If we had a referral from the Salvation Army for instance for someone who is exhibiting psychotic symptoms, so uses street drugs, whatever they may be, we would like to have a system where we could give someone an assessment automatically and have slots where we could give joint assessments from the BSDS and from secondary mental health services. So that's the sort of thinking we're trying to achieve at the moment.

There was an unpublished piece of research I read where one of the people I read who had mental illness compared it to being like a tennis ball, constantly being re referred between BSDS and Community Mental Health Team, and they were wondering, "at what point should I give up asking for help?" This recurred quite a lot in this research paper…

I think unfortunately it does still happen and that's why we want to work more closely with the drugs service. We don't bat people back and forwards between services. What doesn't help is with AWP's undergoing a massive change again and the drugs service is going to be part of a different business unit to Community Mental Health, so we're going to have Trust wide business units for mental health and there's a separate one for drug and alcohol and addiction, so there's even more incentive to try and develop those joint working protocols. It is something we are constantly trying to improve. If you look at our caseload in the inner city the majority have dual diagnosis which speaks for itself really, we don't turn people away. We can't, its part of the reality of working in an Inner City Mental Health Team.

We're constantly trying to improve, there's a long way to go and we'll never stop improving but I think it's really important that we're clear what the issues are.

There is a homeless specialist at the ICMHT and she's off sick.

I'm not sure what this has got to do with your book

What they've found…

Has this come from Margaret Mitchell again?

GIVING VOICE TO THE INNER SCREAM

I want to be helpful to you but I'm actually quite concerned that … this doesn't feel this is about your book

The reason I sit here is because I have found out some stuff which needs to be balanced, all I know is what I have been told, I am not wearing the Salvation Army hat, I want a balanced …

You will appreciate I cannot discuss an individual employee's situation

The reason I ask is that this particular post is not currently operating for some reason or other, be it maternity leave or otherwise and they find there is a degree of difficulty in dealing with ICMHT as a result because that person at the other end of the phone is not there at the moment

I cannot discuss an individual employee's situation. We have a worker in post who works specifically in the homeless sector. Now I feel concerned because this doesn't feel it is about writing a book. This feels like Margaret Mitchell…, and I feel quite uncomfortable with it… It feels like there is another agenda going on here…

The agenda is that I have been told some stuff that needs a response to, because at the end of the day I won a publishing contract and I, if anything I am a broadcast journalist by trade so seek impartiality above all!

I am not suggesting you have another agenda but I am suggesting Margaret Mitchell has another agenda and I think the information she has given you is inaccurate, I think it breaches confidentiality in terms of… staffing, she's not employed by the Trust and I think she has crossed a line really in terms of the information she has given you. I can't really comment any further on that but I do feel concerned at the information she has given you. I am not suggesting you have another agenda but I am suggesting Margaret Mitchell has another agenda.

We have got a worker in post that AWP has funded. The Homeless Mentally Ill Initiative funding was stopped, which came from the Office of the Deputy Prime Minister. Rather than lose that post, which we had identified in one of our reviews, we looked at our skill mix, because we had identified we needed more time with the homeless mentally ill, and we found the resources to fund the post. At the moment it is funded for three days a week but we hope to increase that to full time over time. She has done some fantastic work with the homeless agencies. She's beginning to establish some good relationships and she attends the Homeless Meeting and if you look at what she has achieved with some of the homeless service users and if you look at some of the people who have been passed around and I mean people who have been using drugs and have been excluded from all sorts of accommodation, you know she's done some really good work

GIVING VOICE TO THE INNER SCREAM

I should say that Margaret Mitchell has sung the praises of this woman. To them it meant someone to phone, someone who knew the various issues, and to them life was made a lot easier by having someone there

And she's been in post for a long time, since May, [Interview done in February] and the CAIT team is a single point of referral and in fact all referrals should go through the CAIT team.

Hospital Orders.

Section 117's?

There are a couple of people who have been discharged from Secure Hospitals who are homeless and are known to the SA because they aren't being looked after by the system. This is an extreme version of the 117 Orders that I myself have encountered, where people still have found themselves homeless despite these orders shortly after leaving hospital. Why's this the case?

I can't answer that. The scenario you're presenting. I cannot comment on individual cases. In terms of Section 117, the council and the Trust have a duty for aftercare. We address that through the Integrated Care Programme Approach. If there are cases as you have described they must be brought to the attention of the Trust... via the complaints procedure I guess. I can't comment, we try to follow due process, which is following statutory policy and following Integrated Care Programme Approach [hence, ICPA] *processes.*

Going back to the dial diagnosis tennis ball situation, one final question. How do the teams work together at present? You say you're trying to improve…

We're trying to improve

How do they work together at the moment?

I think it's quite anecdotal and ad hoc. One of the issues that have come to light is that we follow the ICPA process and they do not. So there are different standards and I guess individuals, individual team managers make contact but there are… We did do some work which involved Jerry Monahaghn, Sue Bancroft at the time… It was a few years back … to establish a care pathway and to address that very care pathway you mention and there's a very well established care pathway and a meeting that happens every week in the sector which of course people from the Salvation Army attend. We definitely need some clarity around it and some clear protocols and work was started.

You need this clarity?

We want to avoid being problematic for people to get their needs assessed whether it is for their mental health or drug needs or both so for example the majority of referrals we get are for people with dual diagnosis so we try to set up as many joint assessments as we can but obviously that has got massive issues in terms of resources for each team and hopefully for the strategic business units the Trust has set up the Trust are going to take a lead on this and we can hopefully make sure it is up to service governance and we can get those protocols agreed.

Why doesn't the BSDS not follow the ICPA policy?

No and it is being taken up by the Trust. The Trust states that if people have serious mental illness and a dual diagnosis the ICPA must be followed. The BSDS have their own psychiatrists, their own CPN's, they're geared up to work with people of dual diagnosis as well as the expertise around addiction.

So the BSDS can deal with someone with a major drug problem and a minor mental problem?

It would be helpful to speak to them because they can comment directly on this.

Thank you.

Lynette went on to ask for final approval of this chapter. I refused, though accepted she could have a copy of the questions I put to her. This I revoked on return home, on basis that the interview could be used as ammunition in a strike against the Salvation Army. Instead I have attempted to reproduce the conversation in its best integrity.

Dr Jan Melchiar, Consultant Psychiatrist at the BSDS has his own input into this, saying at the same time that his views do not necessarily represent those of AWP's. Lynette said that the BSDS does not observe the ICPA, and found fault with this. In order to cut through the interdepartmental tribalism that is becoming apparent in the Avon and Wiltshire Partnership NHS Trust, I suggested she had accused the BSDS of not observing this bureaucratic schedule for treatment of psychiatric patients...

With regards to ICPA - I am unsure why you say Lynette Duff 'accuses' BSDS of not following the process. Of course we do not follow the ICPA process, as agreed by the Trust. Our patients are not, unless they have a dual diagnosis, mentally ill, in the sense of needing Mental Health teams to be involved. Therefore, they fall outside of the scope of ICPA, which is designed to ensure that people with mental illnesses get the right treatment (and that the right paperwork is filled in).

Of course, we at BSDS are clear, as is the whole of the Drug and Alcohol services within the Trust, that ICPA, done properly, would be a good thing for patients with mental health issues who are also substance mis-users. We are currently trying to see how this should be tied together in the context of the new ICPA process that the Trust has brought in recently, but what is clear is that:

GIVING VOICE TO THE INNER SCREAM

a) Patients/clients of BSDS not suffering from a mental illness (that needs Mental Health Team input) do not require ICPA.

b) Those that potentially do have a dual diagnosis will, most likely, require an ICPA that will be managed by the Mental Health Team involved, with BSDS being involved only with regards to the substance misuse. At the moment, we are in the process of seeing how the new ICPA process works, in the context of having >20 other Mental Health Teams in the Bristol and S. Gloucestershire area to liaise with.

The fact that clients with ICPA i.e. with dual diagnosis, should be mainly managed by the Mental Health team, follows from the long acknowledged but rarely implemented fact that people with dual diagnosis should have their mental health needs met by the Mental Health teams and not by the Substance Misuse teams. Unfortunately, this is very difficult to actually implement, as BSDS and similar teams continue to be seen as the Substance Misuse 'Mental Health teams', without understanding that we cannot provide or have easy access to psychiatrically-trained staff or out-of-hours care. In essence, we are a '9to5' service that provides long-term care and are not funded or set-up to provide 'crisis' or 'acute' care, which is what Mental Health services generally are. Hence there is sometimes confusion about what our role is.
++++++++++++++++++++

Hence there is sometimes confusion about what our role is[79]

This could be brought in direct comparison to Lynette's

Because generally people without psychosis, people who are treated with depression, are usually managed in primary care.

… I think that's where the tension sits

This is despite

people often reach crisis point before being seen by a mental health team.[80]

One would hope that one day that "confusion" and "tension" are applied solely to the psychiatric service users and drugs mis-users, not the secondary mental health system!

Co ordination is crucial if one of the 90% of the homeless that appear at the Salvation Army in Little George Street with mental health problems and drug addictions, are to get treated effectively and with the minimum fuss. This is not, and apparently cannot be the case with a system full of

---

[79] Repeated deliberately

[80] See Centrepoint article at beginning of this chapter. Alternatively, http://www.centrepoint.org.uk/content/view/183/41/ for the entire article

bottle necks and resistance to taking the people it should care for in the first place.

On receipt of Jan Melchiar's response, I came up with the title of this chapter – *the Basket weavers and the basket case*. Service users famously weave baskets in "Occupational Therapy", giving rise to the derisive term "Basket case". In many respects in order to become a basket weaver in the Inner City area of Bristol you have to deal with a basket case of a mental health admission system.

In Lynette's term; the very small part that Margaret Mitchell plays in the overall scheme, is working very hard to deal with the effect of the *tension* and *confusion* of a system that should be dealing with people's mental health problems whilst not being distracted by its own.

Avon and Wiltshire Partnership NHS Trust is in the midst of a corporate reorganisation that one hopes will have a greater effect than a change in the paper trail from service user to the Chief Executive. One hopes that resources can be found in its vaunted efficiencies to end the interdepartmental "games of tennis" that take place, and perhaps get people treated before they become seriously ill and require far more expense and work than prior to this reorganisation[81].

---

[81] Ibid

For this section I will draw out a final quote from Dr Jan Melchiar which would save the graces of the staff that work within a crazy system that does but reluctantly, treat people that are crazy in their own right.

It is important, though, to remember that all those working in Mental Health and BSDS are trying to do their best!

The last word...

Phewwww! The end of the book. I have often read of the hell that people go through coming up to the submission date of their book. Read Hunter S Thompson's *Kingdom of Fear* for insight from someone Ralph Steadman said was almost incapable of making a deadline in his later years – Steadman foresaw the suicide in a deadline being made quietly for some photos being done and an article being written! [82] I have a slight mood disorder where I go through the highs and lows of living a little more than most so you must appreciate that the writing of this book has had some stellar highs and deep lows...

The least high point was getting the contract in the first place – I never celebrated it in the end. It took 3 hours from the sample chapter going to Chipmunka, and I was convinced that this was a contract to *read* the bloody thing, not the deal itself! The most high was getting a plain white envelope in the post with some work in it from Second Step. Yippee I thought, now an unmarked envelope containing some negotiating documents from a supported housing provider and tomorrow John Prescott's phone logs! So I told Jane Drake thank you and impugned that I would ask for the phone logs of the Deputy PM - and they cut off all contact with me, only I wouldn't ask someone in such a position of trust for this at all, and nearly buggered up writing this book as a result!

---

[82] In *The joke's over*

It has been a journey of understanding. From the day I challenged my own perceptions of the psycho killer and walked through the door of the supported house in Bristol to meet Andrew, I have had to challenge my own perceptions and prejudices in life. Bullshit – I started to challenge perceptions and prejudices at an early age and this has been the culmination of years' work on my own self improvement. I remember for instance the newly anointed Head Boy at school who came and sat with me, on the Rejects' table at school one lunchtime to show his political allegiances were with the lesser man as with the winners of the school. I have always looked for the strength in people and not the rotten outside of them. Bull's pat... I am no one to look up to, I have concealed stuff here that would make anyone blanch, the teenage dope fiending that David Cameron did[83] are some of the things I celebrate, the ones kept silent...? Male cow's dung, somewhere between the above assertions you will find a middle ground.

Writing this book has put to rest two aspects of my personality. I understand my psychosis and it is again a private entity that few will ever hear me speak of. It is unnecessary to speak of mental illness except as abstraction, now I have better things to trade on socially – my MA and this book for instance. It has also been a good while since I needed intoxication in public. Being drunk and full of Dutch courage was something I did as a twenty-

---

[83] One of the many articles...
http://news.independent.co.uk/uk/politics/article2281398.ece

something, and it never really worked anyway. Being sober and sometimes maddeningly sharp in conversation is a far better way to be. Knowing this, I also know that drugs are a necessary part of life for some people and I have a remarkable insight into why. I hope I have imbued this on the reader too!

I don't suggest that the pair of losers who banged an old lady on the head and let her die for the £5 contents of her wallet down the hill from me are forgivable, but will assert that the people I knew as the Odd Couple up the hill from where that happened are more representative of the general junky one finds in the world. They sold everything they possessed for their next heroin fix, and wouldn't hurt a fly for their addiction. One of the Odd Couple was one of the best read, most intelligent people I have ever met, and I have known a few!

No, when you situate George Best and Pete Doherty I want you to see the same man, high or low. I choose these two people because one was celebrated by the mainstream as he drank himself to death and the other was hounded by journalists to the point his mother had to write a book to silence the lies that surrounded her son and family[84].

Through writing this particular chapter, *Junky*, I went through a process of understanding that

---

[84] Jacqueline Doherty (2006) *My prodigal son*

nearly drove me nuts again in doing so. Going through the process highlighted the ugliness I underwent as a maturing addict and son, and where I had lost my way at times. Reading this, Mum and Dad deserve to shoot me for the honesty in it. Some of the things I did, the dishonesty and devilry is something that was very hard to come to terms with in its writing, and proves in my own mind the level of criminality that is involved in the pursuit of a drugs high. My friend Kim Berryman's father went through a tough time on her being incarcerated in a Federal Penitentiary for her methamphetamine addiction; my own parents were exposed to equally unforgivable activities not for 6 years with Kim's addiction, but over 15 with me. Crystal Meth, Junk or fine Port and a Cuban stogie, they're all drugs in the end and the privations you put others through in their pursuit is only of comparison to the other addict. As I apologise to my parents here, so I hope George Bush will apologise for his addiction to God and raising Hell in His Name, and so the nicotine addict will… We're all the same and differentiating between us is not the problem, it is the labelling as "people of choice", and not "enslaved to the drug that masters them".

To the rest of the book again, I want you to equate me with Andrew the psycho killer. Among the readership of this book is one killer who committed murder because of paranoid schizophrenia. He is now less likely to kill than the next man. Because of the stigma of mental illness I am labelled as he even though in the scheme of things he is a safer guy to be around than I am.

I want you to situate Hunter S Thompson with the weirdo who gets pissed on a Friday night and breaks bottles round peoples' heads. Both of them are celebrated for their actions (and occasionally done down in the media). But both should spend some time in a psychiatric unit to cool off, and I have got a psychiatrist to say as much.

On the day the first draft of the Last Word is written, so Robbie Williams has gone into rehab for prescription drug addiction. The forefront paper of the intelligentsia and hero of all paedo's, from 'philes to 'tricians, *The Sun* relates the story[85].

Robbie admitted into rehab

By ONLINE REPORTER
February 13, 2007

ROBBIE WILLIAMS has been admitted into rehab for treatment for his dependency on prescription drugs, his spokeswoman said today.
The former Take That star, who is 33 today, has entered a clinic in the US.
His spokeswoman BRYONY WATTS said: "Robbie Williams has today been admitted into a

---

[85] Have to reference it so here goes, a link to *The Sun* of all places… http://www.thesun.co.uk/article/0,,2004580002-2007070255,00.html?CMP=KNC-powersearchSEM1&HBX_PK=robbie+williams&HBX_OU=50

treatment centre in America for his dependency on prescription drugs.

"There will be no further comment on this matter."

This is not the first time the star, who now lives in LA, has battled with his demons.

After he left Take That, he entered rehab for addiction to drink and drugs.

Model LISA D'AMATO recently revealed Robbie was taking antidepressants and was plagued with worries about his image.

She said: "It was clear he was struggling with his mind. He doesn't drink, but he needs antidepressants to get him through the day. A lot of the time he seemed on edge."

Robbie received mixed reviews for his latest album Rudebox and only one Brit nomination.

He recently cancelled the Asia leg of his Close Encounters world tour, citing stress and exhaustion as the reason.

Just watch and see how everyone in the Celebrity world joins in, relating their own "prescription drugs addiction". There are enough benzo addicts out there so why not come out and admit it like the closet "manic depressives" did after Stephen Fry admitted his illness not long ago…

In two investigations I have highlighted schemes that are trying to lift people and their chaotic lifestyles out of trouble and try to enable them to obey the strictures of society's conventions. To stop being of the stereotyped dribbling, twitchy schizophrenic or even the knife wielding type! Schemes and organisations of this kind are constantly finding difficulty with the State, whether it is funding cuts or institutional stubbornness. Of the options ahead of me as I finish writing this book, I might look at other organisations and schemes in the way of getting people on the rails again (I can think of a few). Second Step and the Salvation Army are but two of many, and sadly there just isn't a body of journalists writing on it as with say the Health Correspondents who focus so heavily on the latest breast cancer drug. Happily for me as I have a market for my writing!

Will you be a better person for reading this? If you learn to deal with everyone with an open mind…? If you don't just label the brainless dickbird with long legs and nice tits on TV as a "dream partner", you will have taken a step in the right direction. I don't say that the bag lady at Paddington Station is more sexually appealing, just that she might have more to say about the world than the leggy blonde airhead. Try it and you might just find out!

RMS, 28/2/07

Appendix – diagnosis suggestions for Hunter S Thompson

This is the original "Diagnosis request" with commentary highlighted in bold italics.

History of the present illness

Robert was expelled from school without matriculating. Jailed in the 1950's for armed robbery, after some years drifting between jobs, he became a journalist. This started a stunning career and he is now a millionaire with a ranch in the Rocky Mountains in the US. **– expelled/robbery – possible conduct disorder/ antisocial personality traits/ perhaps substance misuse / perhaps none of above. Steady career in journalism suggests some stability rather than chaotic lifestyle you might expect with severe antisocial personality disorder/substance misuse problems**

Despite his success, he has had frequent brushes with the law ranging from driving while under the influence to accusations of sexual assault and firearms offences. **He has abused drugs, he is known to drink brandy from first thing in the morning and takes a large amount of illegal narcotics. Sounds like dependent on alcohol and misusing other drugs. Sexual assault charges might be related to substance use (dis-inhibition?), personality (antisocial), or** *could be none of these – e.g. not true, or due to genuine misunderstanding etc...*

He has been married twice and has a son by the first marriage. Family life is good, though friendships and work relationships have been suffering.

Known medical information

He drinks around two litres of brandy per day. He does this from the time he gets up in the morning. He is well known to drink whilst driving. A close friend describes his method for drinking beer, brandy, and smoking marijuana simultaneously whilst at the wheel. **Dependency on alcohol/drugs**

He regularly snorts cocaine. It is known he uses this and other stimulants to start in the morning and uses marijuana and alcohol to help him sleep in the evening. Reports from family and friends suggest that his cocaine abuse is habitual.

In the 1960's and 70's he wrote accounts of taking large doses of hallucinogenic substances ranging from LSD to mescaline to DMT. See, Extract of stream of consciousness account of a drugs trip.

Physical illnesses.

He has had a range of medical problems over the years. Currently he has severe arthritis in his hands, and whole body shakes uncontrollably for reasons unknown. **Presumably related to alcohol/drug misuse**

Psychology

Robert has a persistent belief that the US Federal authorities will storm his house. Has had slam shut gates installed on driveway to home for protection and has an arsenal of firearms. **Any genuine reason for this – e.g. has he committed any offences/been implicated in any offences that would warrant such a belief. If absolutely no justification for this then suggests persecutory ideas that might be due to substance misuse/withdrawal, or unrelated to substances (but one would imagine former more likely given his history so far) – unable to tell without long period of detox and assessment.**

Temper volatile at best, prone to violent rages. People feel unsafe around him at times. **Could be substance use related (most likely), personality traits**

Has extreme political views. Hates neo-conservatism to an unusual degree. See Letter to editor of the UK Independent newspaper.

Destruction of own and others' property – use of TNT and plastic explosives at home to destroy property, likes to hunt and shoot animals for pleasure (**as do many people – possibly** *sadistic/antisocial traits* **BUT more likely could just be what most would consider normal behaviour, e.g. fox hunting, etc....)** *Leaves hotel rooms in unusable state after vacating them.* **Suggests either he is intoxicated, or doesn't care – latter again would suggest some antisocial traits**

Use of firearms. Prone to pointing a high powered handgun in peoples' faces in fit of temper unpleasant – **could be substance use related, personality related... Fascination with weaponry bordering on obsessional – very concerning but impossible to suggest possible reasons (though such fascinations are seen in people with paranoid traits/psychotic illnesses sometimes).** *Recites the US Constitution to reinforce.*

Sometimes incapable of making engagements, personal or otherwise, at times. Missed a Mohammed Ali fight in Zaire and a UK royal engagement despite being flown to both and being paid well. **Most likely seems substance use related – though again maybe just doesn't care (personality). There are always other possibilities for any of behaviours so far (e.g. very depressed and couldn't get out of bed, or very obsess ional and couldn't stop checking that the doors were locked! – but nothing so far suggests any of these or other possibilities)**

Sleep patterns non existent and unpredictable. May sleep all night and work all day or the reverse. **Most likely due to substance use**

Relationships

Work.

Robert is an extremely talented writer in high demand by a range of publications worldwide surprising in view of level of substance misuse and history so far. Has several factual and fiction books published. He is egocentric and proud of his achievements.

However his unpredictability and behaviour makes working with him extremely difficult at times substance use perhaps or personality traits **could be that he is uncaring/cold, or perhaps too obsess ional, or too pessimistic etc....** *Sometimes he makes a print deadline with minutes to spare, at others this is not achieved.*

His paymasters accept this as par for the course but dislike working with him – his name sells papers and magazines so have to put up with it for circulation.

Social relationships

Again, people are drawn to the legend of the man but repelled by the behaviour and unpredictability.

GIVING VOICE TO THE INNER SCREAM

People are drawn to the unpredictability because it is fun but often this has had near fatal consequences – a close friend recounts drink driving and narcotic abuse situations that were frightening at the time but were "good to talk about in the pub after".

Prone to telling people to leave and never return from his life and then blame them for not contacting him. **Blaming others for ones own problems tends to be a feature in antisocial personality disorder, but is also seen in many other situations – we all blame others sometimes though saying to leave one's life is quite extreme, but it is really more the pervasive nature that is characteristic of antisocial behaviour. Also could be seen as an emotionally unstable personality trait – again the role of substance misuse here is not clear – e.g. maybe says this when very intoxicated and then has no recall of ever having said it (so understandably blaming others for not contacting him!)**

Personal relationships

Robert has been married twice. Both were comfortable marriages, no remarked upon violence against the spouses. However he is a sexual predator and has had a string of affairs during this time. He was accused of rape but this was put down by the Courts to a malicious accusation. **Severe antisocial personality disorder usually unable to maintain** *relationships – 2 comfortable marriages doesn't really sound like that. Of course milder antisocial traits may still be present – however most people who have 2 failed marriages and a string of affairs would not be classed as antisocial. The accusations of rape suggest perhaps antisocial personality traits but again could be related to substance use (perhaps most likely) or neither*

++++++++++++++++++++

Printed in the United Kingdom
by Lightning Source UK Ltd.
R751700001B/R7517PG123353UKX1B/1-30/9